GI Janel

Permanent IBS/SIBO Resolution

Table of Contents

Printed in the United States of America

First Printing, 2019

ISBN 978-1-7330562-0-5

GI Janel, Inc

Specialty Natural Medicine, Inc PC

8423 Mukilteo Speedway, Suite 101

Mukilteo WA, 98275

GIJanel.com

SpecialtyNaturalMedicine.com

This book is not intended as a substitute for the medical advice of physicians. The reader should regularly consult a physician in matters relating to his/her health and particularly with respect to any symptoms that may require diagnosis or medical attention.

1 OVERVIEW

Small Intestinal Bacterial Overgrowth (SIBO) is not the cause of your symptoms. Irritable Bowel Syndrome (IBS) is not the cause of your symptoms.

SIBO and IBS are a result of GI (gastrointestinal) Barrier Breakdown, Chronic Inflammatory Response, Food Intolerance and System Deficiency.

If these causes are not addressed, symptoms can and will easily return even after antibiotic treatment. The GI Janel system works to repair the GI barrier (gastrointestinal barrier), resolve local motility, reduce inflammation, and support system deficiency. All you need to do is remove your unique irritating foods, then gradually add them back once you are stronger. You do not need to undertake long-term, complexed diet restrictions.

IBS and SIBO are typically not the result of any single cause. Therefore, no single magic bullet treatment has successfully been developed to resolve them.

IBS and SIBO are *functional disorders*, in that the function of the digestive system is compromised and must be addressed at all levels of digestive deterioration for symptom relief.

The first SIBO testing came out in the 1990's. I have been using this test and other functional medicine testing that you will learn about in this book for over two decades. As a result, I have accumulated a vast amount of knowledge and clinical experience in functional digestive medicine. I have developed a unique approach to the resolution of IBS and SIBO that I will take you through in this book, providing the steps that you can follow to relieve your own symptoms.

After successfully treating Irritable Bowel Syndrome and Small Intestinal Bacterial Overgrowth (IBS/SIBO) for over 20 years, I can confidently say that there is no need for anyone to live with their symptom, to continue long term restrictive diets or to expect a symptom relapse.

2 CONSULTATIONS FOR IBS/SIBO

In this book, I have attempted to provide all the material you will need to resolve your symptoms of IBS (Irritable bowel syndrome), SIBO (small intestinal bacterial overgrowth) and SIFO (small intestinal fungal overgrowth) with my line of supplements, GI Janel.

For advanced treatment or questions, I recommend that you contact us at GI Janel Anywhere. Some patients will require additional diagnostics or advanced treatment in terms of natural or prescription therapy which is beyond the scope of this book. You can apply for a consultation by visiting consult.gijanel.com and completing the intake information.

We can do remote telemedicine visits in order to answer questions to personalize your treatment experience. We can recommend further supplement intervention through our online pharmacy. We can also support dietary questions and help coach you in the nuances of your personal treatment successes.

My clinic is located just north of Seattle, Washington. Together, our support team and associates have developed an environment where we take the time to listen to our patients, coach them and provide the best care we can while integrating natural and prescriptive medicines. We provide additional core treatments to strengthen the body. This includes intravenous (IV) nutrient therapy, visceral (digestive) massage, bio-puncture (natural pain management), food and allergy desensitization. While I specialize in digestive disorders, my associates provide family medicine and specialize in integrative endocrinology, pediatric care and chronic disease.

I look forward to taking this healing journey with you and I want you to be well,

Dr Kathleen Janel & the GI Janel Team.

SpecialtyNaturalMedicine.com

Consult.GIJanel.com

IBS and SIBO are Functional Defects. They can be diagnosed, treated and resolved.

3 Introduction, Why GI Janel Works

~ There will always be more answers.

I wrote this book because I have witnessed remarkable success with my patients when they use my plan to resolve their digestive issues. What I am sharing in this book is a unique approach to the permanent resolution of digestive symptoms. It is a different approach from what you are hearing from other functional medical doctors. For over 20 years I have been refining my approach in the treatment of digestive symptoms. What I am offering you here is what I have come to understand.

My approach will be different than what you may learn from other functional doctors and gastroenterologists. This is because I found a way to treat IBS and SIBO many years ago and have continued to use this approach, refining it over the years. I do not advocate long term dietary restrictions or the long-term use of natural or prescription antibiotics, and yet have had hundreds of successful cases (sometimes very quickly). I focus on strengthening the digestive system and achieving homeostasis in the microbiome. I wrote this book so that I could help provide resolution for those struggling to find relief while doing everything they can, yet not seeing progress or relapsing over and over.

IBS/SIBO are functional disorders arising from chronic inflammation in the digestive system, from intestinal cell damage, nutrient depletion, and the inappropriate interface of the immune system with the digestive contents.

When the intestinal cells are not healthy, they cannot effectively participate in their major functions. Results include failure to fully break down food for absorption and the failure to provide an effective Gastrointestinal barrier that separates immune cells from the products of digestion.

The GI Janel system addresses the underlying reasons for the development of Irritable Bowel Syndrome, Small Intestinal Bacterial Overgrowth, Small Intestinal Fungal Overgrowth and

Dysbiosis. It strengthens the digestive system and allows the body to come back into a strong homeostasis (balance).

SIBO (small intestinal bacterial overgrowth) occurs when normal or abnormal bacteria overgrow in the small intestine, allowing them to use your food for fuel before you can digest it. When these bacteria use your food for their own fuel, they produce excess gas. You become bloated and possibly in great pain with abdominal distention.

SIFO (small intestinal fungal overgrowth) is like SIBO, but fungal species predominate. SIFO and SIBO can occur together or separately. Endoscopic studies carried out by Dr. Satish C. Rao have determined that 25% of people with gas and bloating have SIFO, 35% have SIBO and 40% have mixed SIBO and SIFO. He has determined that 90% of the fungal species are Candida. There can also be overgrowth of either yeast of unwanted bacteria in the large intestine. This is called dysbiosis (bad microbiome).

IBS (Irritable Bowel Syndrome) can occur with SIBO/SIFO or it can be independent. It can include the symptoms of gas and bloating and pain that are signatures of SIBO/SIFO. These can be in addition to other problems that may or may not stem from SIBO, such as constipation, diarrhea, nausea, and cramping pains. IBS and SIBO/SIFO can be addressed together for full symptom resolution because the underlying causes are the same. They are functional problems (action or physiology problems) in which the anatomy can appear normal on scopes (colonoscopy or endoscopy) and imaging.

IBS is different from the other very common digestive disease called IBD (Inflammatory Bowel Disease). IBD can be life threatening due to the severity of symptoms. It includes Crohn's disease and Ulcerative Colitis. Symptoms primarily mimic those of IBS-D (IBS Diarrhea dominant) with the addition of debilitating diarrhea and fluid loss, bleeding, mucous production and severe painful inflammation which can be detected on GI scopes with biopsies. IBD is a functional and an anatomical problem with a genetic influence.

I have a very personal history with digestive symptoms. In fact, I was at the height of discomfort during my premed education. My own gas, bloating and severe pain were so intense that even drinking water would bring symptoms on. I lost a dangerous amount of weight because of the pain associated with eating any food. After some testing was done which turned out normal, there really were no more answers for me from my doctors. During that time, I was focused on my applications for medical school and I had absolutely no intention of becoming an alternative doctor. I had made up my mind that anything off the beaten track of conventional medicine was not for me. You can imagine then, the reluctance I had to see a naturopathic doctor when a friend recommended that I try this approach. But I was desperate for relief.

This doctor changed my diet, gave me supplements to take and I immediately began to feel better. My suspicion of alternative medicine was being challenged by my own experience. I decided to send applications into both naturopathic medical school and to conventional medical school that year. When I was accepted at both, I had a big decision to make! Do I take the well-traveled route or the fork in the road? I had some heated conversations with my friends who did not understand why I was even considering an alternative to conventional medical school. But I had to do it. I had to understand how to help my patients like that first Naturopathic Doctor helped me. The choice I made continues to be rewarding. I attended a four-year post graduate doctoral program at Bastyr University to become a Naturopathic Doctor (ND) and went on to complete a two-year residency position in integrative medicine.

In Washington State and some others, NDs are considered primary care providers and we can prescribe pharmaceutical medicine along with natural medicines, lifestyle modifications and dietary treatments.

The first test I used for SIBO detection came out in the early 1990's. It has become more well-known over time and more widely available for the detection of bacterial overgrowth in the small intestine. SIBO is one part of the picture in a complexed system. Addressing SIBO with antibiotics alone, whether natural or pharmaceutical, rarely achieves permanent resolution of horrible digestive symptoms.

The results I have seen over and over have convinced me that digestive problems including gas, bloating, pain, nausea, diarrhea, reflux and constipation do not have to be what you live with. The people whom I treat come from all over. Many have discovered my clinic after seeing other doctors or attempting their own treatments with only short-term success or no improvement at all.

Just recently I treated a young woman who came into see me following two years of worsening digestive symptoms. She had been given a diagnosis of functional dyspepsia which essentially means her system is functioning in a way that causes indigestion. She had lost over 25 lbs. because everything she ate gave her severe digestive symptoms. The symptoms began after a trip to Mexico two years prior. She had seen a gastroenterologist and had a normal endoscopy (EGD) and a normal colonoscopy. All her other testing and blood work was also normal.

Her stools were burning, and she felt a burning sensation in her digestive system as food moved through her. She would have constipation and then diarrhea, bloating, pain and burning, smelly gas. She had tried low carbohydrate diets, Fodmap diet, Ketogenic diet (high fat) diet and several over the counter digestive supplements but nothing changed her symptoms.

We began by collecting samples for food intolerances and digestive overgrowth. I started her on GI Janel One powder and my soft food diet while we were waiting for the results. Four weeks later, we met again to review her lab results and she reported that her symptoms had already improved. She was astonished and hopeful. At that point, I asked her to begin to eat more of a variety of soft foods that were negative on her intolerance test and I asked her to increase her dose of GI Janel One powder gradually to six teaspoons a day.

She returned four weeks later to let me know that all her symptoms resolved once she reached 3 teaspoons on GI Janel One. At her follow up visit with me ten months later, she was continuing her soft food diet and avoiding her known triggers (Dairy and Gluten) but had re-introduced all other food. She stayed on a maintenance dose of GI Janel One powder of 1 tsp per day. Her symptoms continue to be resolved.

This example of resolution is a very quick one, but it is not unusual. I see several cases like this every year.

I have seen frustrated people who have been told that there is nothing wrong with them, who have been told that their diet has nothing to do with their digestive symptoms, who have been told that they are imagining their symptoms or that their symptoms are caused by depression.

Twenty years ago, I even had patients telling me that their GI doctor told them that there are no bacteria that live in their digestive system. We've come a long way since then.

My personal health history involved much research and testing to alleviate my own daily, debilitating (and embarrassing) bloating, pain, diarrhea, nausea, constipation and heartburn. Because of this, in the early days of treating my patients, I would experiment along with them, differentiating what sounded good in theory but clinically did little to resolve symptoms, or even made them worse. This was twenty years ago, and my symptoms have never returned. I am free to eat whatever I like.

I have seen treatments come and go and have seen our diagnostic skills in functional medicine grow as we understand and incorporate more knowledge. We are always learning. However, I came to understand very early on in my practice that the treatment of IBS/SIBO can require some focused dietary changes that are unique to everyone. These diet changes are teamed with regenerative supplements in the GI Janel treatment plan.

Following my protocol will lead to decreased inflammation, increased strength and improved function of the digestive system. You will then be able to tolerate many foods again without symptoms. My goal is for you to eventually eat what you want without having to think about it.

I want success for my patients. I want the permanent elimination of digestive issues along with the ability to have an unrestrictive diet. This led me to develop the unique supplements that I have seen work effectively, time and time again for my patients over the course of the past two decades.

I am writing this book for all those people who have digestive symptoms of IBS/SIBO and must deal with the inconvenience and discomfort of this on an ongoing basis.

I am writing this for the people who have given up and have decided to just live with their symptoms.

I am writing this book for those people who are trying their best and the plan is just not working to provide permanent relief. I am writing this book for all of you who have used ongoing restrictive diets because at best they give you some relief.

I am here to tell you that if you resolve the chronic inflammation, regenerate the health of your digestive cells and allow your body's immune system to recover its strength, your symptoms will resolve, and you will no longer have to eliminate foods from your diet.

4 INNATE WISDOM

Listen to your body when it whispers, so you won't have to hear it scream.

---Author Unknown

The core principle of my medical practice is that your body has an innate healing intelligence. This intelligence knows what is needed to keep you healthy, vital and thriving. In medical school, we refer to this the *Vital Force*.

This is part of the oath we take as graduating physicians:

The Healing Power of Nature:

We recognize an inherent self-healing process in people that is ordered and intelligent. As physicians, we act to identify and remove obstacles to healing and recovery, and to facilitate and augment this inherent self-healing process.

The mechanism of this healing force is expressed in the form of trillions of chemical and electrical reactions happening inside of you without you having to even think about it. However, when the vital force is constantly irritated by something in your environment (internal or external), it can weaken.

The primary language that represents the vitality of the body's innate intelligence is the immune system. The immune system's job is to protect you from infections that cause disease. The immune system is a vital component of the innate wisdom that keeps you alive and strong.

Here's an example. Did you know that every day your body is producing cancer cells? These cells cannot join forces and lump together to become cancer tumors because you have an immune system that is constantly tracking and destroying these cells. [1]

The vital force weakens if it is constantly irritated (by chronic infections and irritations, including food intolerances) or when it is deficient in nutrient supply for building and maintaining the body (lack of nutrients). The body will first begin to express the problem as acute symptoms related directly to the irritation (like colic pain or vomiting in a baby who is exposed to a food it is not ready for). These symptoms can increase over time if the problem irritation is not addressed.

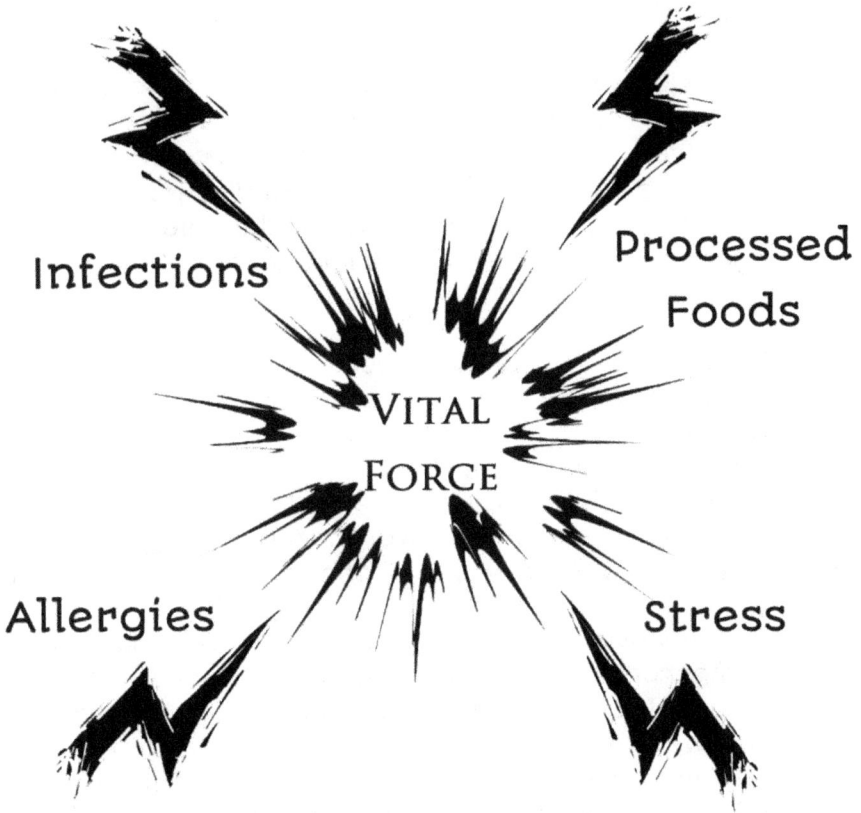

Figure 4.1 Constant Irritations shrink the Vital Force (immune system)

In addition to the acute symptoms expressed by the body, over time, the immune system begins to take a toll because of ongoing irritation and insult. Then, the weakness of the immune system begins to express itself. For example, if a baby's body is not ready for cow dairy, yet continues to have it, we can see symptoms of immune dysfunction such as chronic tonsillitis, chronic ear infection, difficult teething episodes, frequent colds or other serious infections.

Babies in my practice that have a controlled and analytic food introduction (including what the mom eats while nursing), rarely have these problems. If I treat a baby who is having these issues and we remove the offending foods and support the developing immune system, the majority return to the state of a thriving infant again. I have written more about this in the Infant Food Introduction chapter.

There is always a reason for your symptoms. Your body is always communicating with you. Symptoms are a message from your body that it needs you to pay attention.

In the case of IBS/SIBO, when we find out what the problem is and solve it, symptoms resolve, and the body heals. This allows us to return to a place where we can eat without major restrictions.

In other disease states, there can be an autoimmune component. Autoimmune means that the body is attacking itself. In autoimmune disease, the innate wisdom is still operating, however the system has lost its ability to tell the difference between what is self and what is non-self. The immune system begins to attack its own body. This occurs in Inflammatory Bowel Disease (Crohn's, Ulcerative Colitis). Because of the complexity of autoimmune gastrointestinal diseases and the severity of symptoms, sometimes the only method to keep the body alive is to suppress the immune system with steroids or the more recent biologic treatments. This does not mean that there are not triggers or some reason that the autoimmune process began, it only means we don't know what the cause or causes are yet. For Crohn's and Ulcerative colitis, the causes are even more complicated as they seem to be a result of a triad that includes genetic, immune and Infectious etiologies (causes).

If it's a matter of life or death or the patient is in severe discomfort, then I strongly support suppressing the immune system with steroids or biologics and I believe that we are fortunate to have these suppressive treatments as an option. However, I also believe at that it is important to continue exploring and researching the reasons for the development of the symptoms so that treatment options can be made available to eventually mitigate damage without weakening the entire immune system with the treatment.

There are two primary functions of the immune system. The most obvious is its protective role. The cells and chemicals of the immune system are continually surveying body and protecting us from infections. They are also busy destroying any cells that may be becoming malignant (cancerous). This is important. Everyone's immune system is operating at a unique capacity and this is dependent on their constitution and history. For example, if you are in an elevator with 10 other people and one person is infectious with a cold virus who then sneezes, you have all been exposed to the virus. However, not everyone in the elevator will be affected by the virus and develop the cold. The simple difference is the strength of one immune system over another (and of course, concentration of viral exposure).

The second and equally important role of the immune system is that of tolerance. We need the immune system cells to tell the difference between a protein on an infectious bacterium versus the protein in a food that we are eating. If the immune system does not recognize the normal internal and external environment and considers them foreign, it will mount an attack on the body or environment. This is the definition of auto immune disease and allergies. Allergy and autoimmune disease are states that lack tolerance to the normal environments. The immune system is attempting to protect us from non-problematic elements of ourselves and the world we live in. Allergies are a lack of tolerance to the outside world

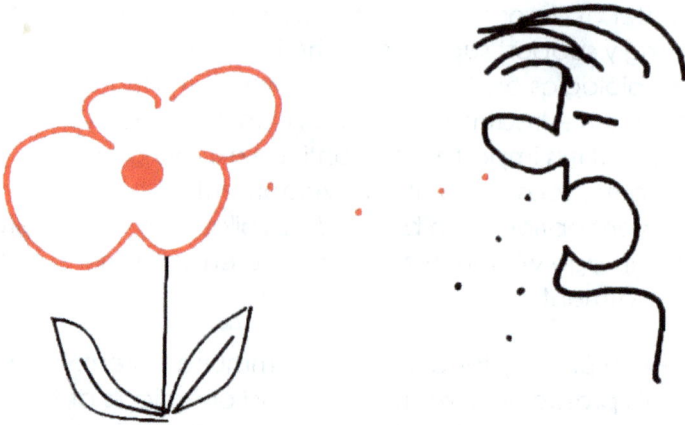

Figure 4.2 *Pollen, a naturally occurring product of plants, can cause a histamine release (sneezing) when the body's tolerance to the pollen is lost.*

Autoimmune disorders are lack of tolerance to self. An example of an autoimmune trigger occurs in the case of rheumatic fever following strep throat. Proteins on the Strep bacteria can mimic proteins in the body, causing the immune system to attack the body thinking the bacteria is still there.

Symptoms do not just randomly happen. Therefore, we want to discover and eliminate the cause of the symptoms so that the immune force can reacquire its strength. A weakened vital force leads to a weakened immune system, which then makes the body more susceptible to disease.

For example, when the body is infected by a virus such as HIV, the immune system is weakened, and the body becomes more susceptible to other viral, bacterial and fungal infections. Therefore, people who carry the HIV virus acquire more infections such as fungal overgrowth in their mouths and lungs and viral skin infections than someone without the HIV virus.

Here's another example. If you eat too many cherries, eventually you will get diarrhea (the symptoms). Eating some is okay, but too many overtax the digestion and loosen the bowels. You can either continue eating the cherries and take a medication to stop the diarrhea, or you can stop eating the cherries.

This may seem like a silly example, but many foods that we eat can be irritating when we have digestive symptoms. Some of those foods are very delicious like gluten, dairy and sugar, but for many people, when we take them away, symptoms improve. Because food reactions can be immediate or delayed, the foods must be removed from the diet for at least two weeks before symptoms start to settle down.

When we can detect and remove irritants that are weakening the vital force, and provide missing nutrients to support weakened systems, your body can then recover its strength and use its healing abilities to make you strong and symptom-free again.

This can occur very quickly once we know what the irritants are. You must be willing to temporarily remove some irritant foods that are unique to you while the repair occurs inside. In this way, we are working with the innate wisdom of the body, and allowing it to strengthen, rather than suppressing symptoms.

The most important message of this book is that IBS and SIBO can be resolved using gentle nutrient-based medicine. The treatment for IBS and SIBO have small, unique variations from person to person, but the result that I've seen for my patients over the past 20 years is that you can live your life without onerous dietary restrictions or disruptive treatments and be free of IBS/SIBO symptoms.

Once the function of the digestive tract is addressed and healed, your body can then carry on and digest your food without symptoms.

The fact that it is NOT carrying on this beautiful orchestration of the digestive process, silently and easily, is your body telling you that it needs a change.

As we go through the treatments in this book, we'll identify what your body requires to resolve your symptoms.

This book has a personal significance to me because I intimately know the discomfort of living with gas, bloating, diarrhea, constipation and chronic abdominal pain. For years I searched for answers, before having complete resolution and the freedom in my diet to eat whatever I want, whenever I want.

I want this for you too.

When my personal IBS/SIBO symptoms were at their worst, even drinking water caused me to have abdominal pain. This seemed ridiculous and even unbelievable. But my experience benefits you. When I have a patient sitting in my exam room claiming a degree of sensitivity like this, I am listening.

5 IBS/ SIBO Defined

~ IBS is a complex, multifunctional disorder.

Irritable bowel syndrome and SIBO (small intestinal bacterial overgrowth) comprise a complex of disorders that manifest in a variety of symptoms. Patients describe any combination of symptoms including abdominal pain, gas, bloating, constipation, diarrhea or alternating constipation and diarrhea. They can also experience nausea. For women, symptoms often worsen around the time of the menstrual period.

SIBO occurs when normal or abnormal bacteria overgrow in the small intestine, allowing them to use your food for fuel before you can digest it. When these bacteria use your food for their own fuel, they produce excess gas. You become bloated and possibly in great pain with abdominal distention.

SIFO (small intestinal fungal overgrowth) is like SIBO, but fungal species predominate. SIFO and SIBO can occur together or separately. Endoscopic studies carried out by Dr. Satish C. Rao have determined that 25% of people with gas and bloating have SIFO, 35% have SIBO and 40% have mixed SIBO and SIFO. He has determined that 90% of the fungal species are Candida.[2] There can also be overgrowth of either yeast of unwanted bacteria in the large intestine. This is called *dysbiosis* (bad microbiome).

IBS (Irritable Bowel Syndrome) can occur with SIBO/SIFO or it can be independent. It can include the symptoms of gas, bloating, and pain that are signatures of SIBO/SIFO. These can be in addition to other problems that may or may not stem from SIBO, such as constipation, diarrhea, nausea, and cramping pains. IBS and SIBO/SIFO can be addressed together for full symptom resolution because the underlying causes are the same. They are functional problems (action or physiology problems) in which the anatomy can appear normal on scopes (colonoscopy or endoscopy) and imaging.

Some IBS/SIBO patients also have separate but related symptoms like reflux (heartburn), gastritis, digestive valve defects or weakness, diverticular disease or hemorrhoids. Often a person's symptoms have no obvious correlation to diet or will happen only when food is eaten. For others the symptoms are continuous or worsen throughout the day and for still others there are periods of flares and remissions.

Although these symptoms are not immediately life threatening, they are disruptive in day to day life and can eventually contribute to other disease states as the body attempts to compensate for the chronic digestive stress. The symptoms will cause discomfort and disruption during the waking hours and pain and insomnia at night for some individuals. IBS and SIBO are also a common part of the symptom picture for people with Chronic Fatigue Syndrome, Biotoxin Disease, Fibromyalgia, Multiple Chemical Sensitivities, Histamine Intolerance and Mast Cell Activation Syndromes.

IBS and SIBO are typically not the result of any single cause. Therefore, no single magic bullet treatment has successfully been developed to resolve them.

They are disorders where the function of the digestive system is compromised. Restoring function must be addressed at all levels of digestive deterioration for symptom relief.

The digestive system is a complex orchestration of chemistry and movement. The food you eat moves food through the intestines. As it moves, it is broken down into smaller and smaller pieces until it is the smallest it can be (the microscopic building block of foods). It can then be absorbed through the cell of the small intestine and enter the body. Whatever remains in the intestine is moved out of the body as waste material through the large intestine. There are many distinct structures and functions through the digestive tract which can play a role in IBS/SIBO symptoms. This is the reason that finding a single drug approach to managing IBS/SIBO symptoms is so difficult, if not impossible.

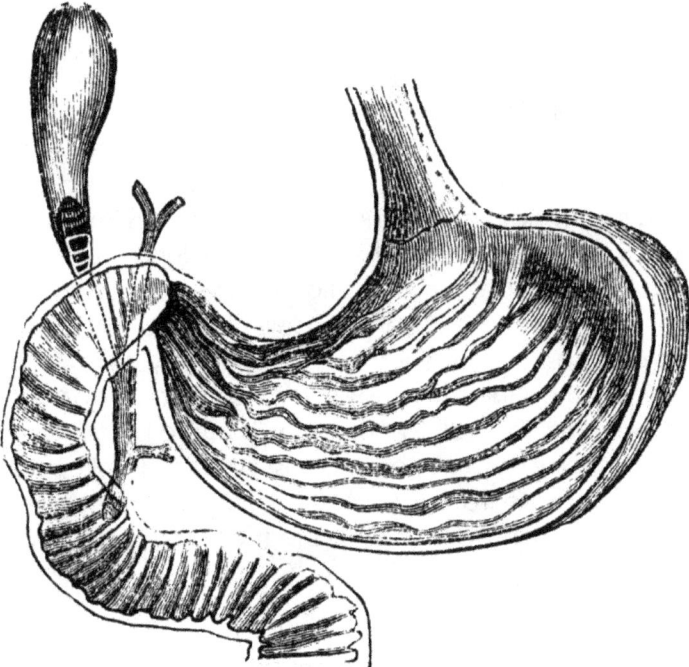

Figure 5.1 As food moves through the digestive system, it is broken down into smaller and smaller pieces.

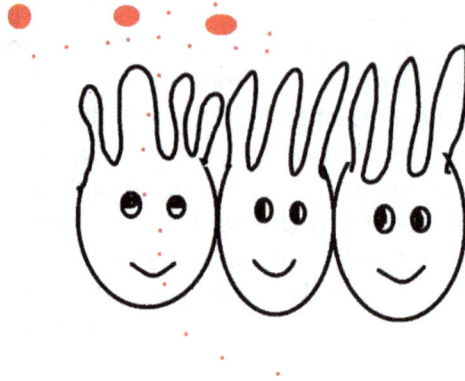

Figure 5.2 *Intestinal cells transport food into the body.*

The first level that must be addressed to alleviate the symptoms of IBS/SIBO is the health of the intestinal cells. The cells of the intestine form a tube. The inside of this tube is called the lumen. I begin treatment here at the cellular level. It is imperative to have healthy intestinal cells forming a healthy lumen and brush border. These intestinal cells must be tightly joined together so that food is selectively moved through the cells and into the body. What nutrients cross from the lumen into the body is therefore dependent on the health of the intestinal cells and the luminal environment. The cell-to-cell tube structure is called the *Gastrointestinal barrier,* and it must be intact to keep the immune system separate from the intestinal (luminal) contents. It also must be strong and intact to complete the final breakdown of food.

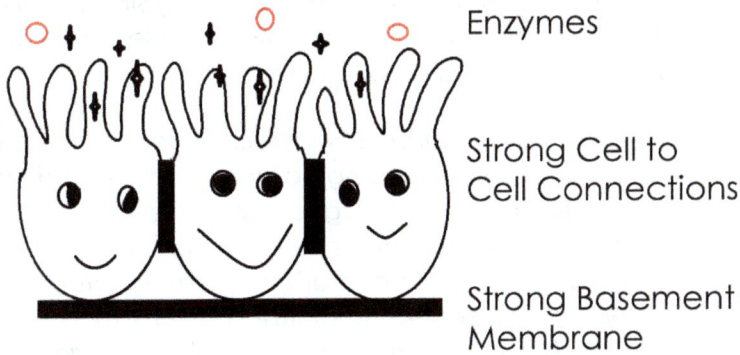

Enzymes

Strong Cell to
Cell Connections

Strong Basement
Membrane

Figure 5.3 *A healthy gastrointestinal barrier separates undigested food in the intestine from the immune system of the body. It has complete cell to cell connections, a strong basement membrane and healthy cells that can release enzymes to complete the final stage of digestion. They also provide a place for the good bacteria to thrive.*

If the gastrointestinal barrier is compromised, the immune system begins fighting foods that you've eaten, and overgrowth of bacterial and fungal species can occur. This creates the gas and bloating discomfort experienced in SIBO/SIFO. When you are gassy, it is not you that is making the gas. That is impossible. The gas is coming from bacteria or yeast that are eating your food and producing copious amounts of methane, hydrogen and hydrogen sulfide gases.

Post infectious SIBO arises following an acute digestive illness, typically food poisoning. The current theory is that the migrating motor complex (MMC) which is your intestinal cleaning system, becomes damaged and the resulting stagnation allows bacterial overgrowth. The migrating motor complex is responsible for cleaning the digestive system. It sweeps residual, undigested food out of the system between meals. This is a housekeeping function. It exists in order to prevent stagnation and overgrowth of bacteria in the intestine. While I have seen the onset of post infections SIBO reported by many patients, I don't use the MMC as the starting point for my treatment. Again, if the cells that form the gastrointestinal barrier are not healthy, no amount of motility regeneration or treatment will prevent relapsing SIBO symptoms. If the health of the cells of the gastrointestinal barrier is repaired, the MMC also returns to its proper rhythm.

> *Here's an example from my practice. I treated a young woman who was attending college in Boston and was referred to me by a colleague practicing there. She reported generalized digestive pain that could be at times dull, achy, sharp or cramping. Her symptoms all started with an episode of diarrhea several months previous. Her symptoms then turned to alternating diarrhea and constipation (IBS-M) with gas, bloating and gas pains (SIBO). Her GI doctor in Boston had given her dicyclomine for spasms and suggested that she follow the low FODMAP diet, which helped a little.*

> *I removed dairy and gluten and gave her a soft food diet to follow while we did food intolerance testing. At her four week follow up visit, she reported more regular stools from using the GI Janel One powder. She had determined that rice, oats, sugar, corn, dairy and gluten or anything with high fiber caused severe bloating. I assured her that this is normal for the course of her treatment and asked her to avoid high fiber and the foods from her intolerance panel, while increasing her dose of the GI Janel One.*

> *By the time we talked again, she was back in Boston for the school year, so we had a visit by phone. She sounded happy, and reported that she was having regular, daily bowel movements, substantially decreased digestive pain and little to no gas or gas pain. She had added fibers back to her diet, including nuts, rice and corn. Since her food panel showed reactions to gluten and dairy, I encouraged her to keep these out of her diet for the next two years. She was going to try oats next in the form of oatmeal and I encouraged her to do this but do it by adding small amounts at a time so that the food could be used as a pre-biotic and coax the growth of her improving microbiome rather than overwhelm it. I suggested that she continue a maintenance dose of GI Janel One and that she continues taking GI Janel Digest B with her meals to provide additional support to her system as it regains its full strength and vitality.*

6 THE INTESTINAL CELL AND IBS/SIBO

~It's all about the GI Barrier

In order to lay the foundational understanding for my treatment plan to resolve IBS/SIBO, I first need to walk you through some basic anatomy and physiology of the digestive system. First, I want to explain how nutrients are transported from the intestinal tube or digestive tract into the body. There are three macronutrients and many micronutrients that are transported. The three macronutrients are: proteins, carbohydrates, and fats. The micronutrients in foods are minerals and vitamins.

The smallest carbohydrate to reach the intestinal cell is the disaccharide. The intestinal cell can transport only monosaccharide building blocks into the body. Each food type: carbohydrates, proteins and fats have building blocks that are small enough to cross the gastrointestinal barrier.

6.1 PROTEIN

Proteins are built from amino acids. There are 20 distinct amino acid building blocks that combine in diverse ways to form all the protein structure in our body. (Isn't that amazing?). The healthy intestinal cell releases protein breaking enzymes called protease from its brush border to break linked amino acids into single amino acids so that they can cross through the gastrointestinal barrier.

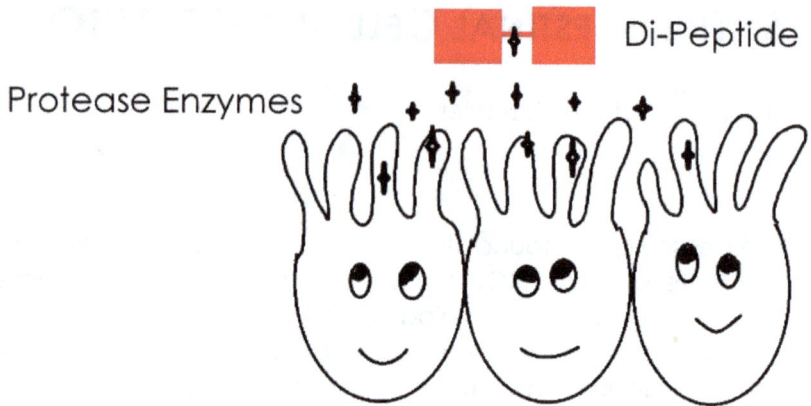

Figure 6.1 *Healthy intestinal cells release proteases for the breakdown of di-peptides in to the smallest building blocks of proteins called amino acids.*

6.2 CARBOHYDRATES (SUGARS)

Carbohydrates are built from monosaccharides. There are three monosaccharides:

- Fructose (fruit sugar)
- Glucose (our main body fuel)
- Galactose (found in animal dairy)

Note that glucose can be taken into the body without further breakdown and used immediately (because it is a monosaccharide).

Disaccharides must be broken into their components before they can enter the intestinal cell. For example, sucrose (table sugar, typically cane sugar) is broken into its components, glucose and fructose. There are three disaccharides:

- Sucrose (table sugar or cane sugar)
- Lactose (milk sugar)
- Maltose (starchy foods)

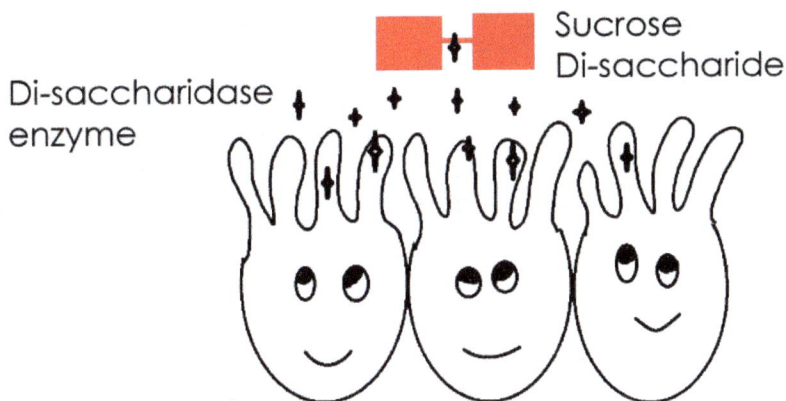

Di-saccharidase enzyme

Sucrose Di-saccharide

Figure 6.2 *Table sugar (sucrose) is split into glucose and fructose monosaccharides, which can then be transported across the gastrointestinal barrier.*

Fructose (because it is a monosaccharide) can also be absorbed directly by the intestinal cell, but it must be converted by the liver into either fat or glucose for the body to use it. Can you see here the problem with high fructose corn syrup products? They are made from highly concentrated fructose that will turn to fat in the liver if the body has enough glucose already available. This is not the same as eating a piece of fruit which contains substantially less fructose and contains fiber to slow the absorption of the fructose. The explosion of NAFLD (nonalcoholic fatty liver disease) is directly related to our over consumption of sugars that the liver turns into fat. [3]

6.3 FAT

Fats are built from glycerol and fatty acids chains. One glycerol is attached to three fat chains to make a fat. That is why fats are called *triglycerides* (the *tri* refers to the three fat chains). They are also referred to as *triacyl glycerides* or TAGs. These show up on your cholesterol panel as triglycerides.

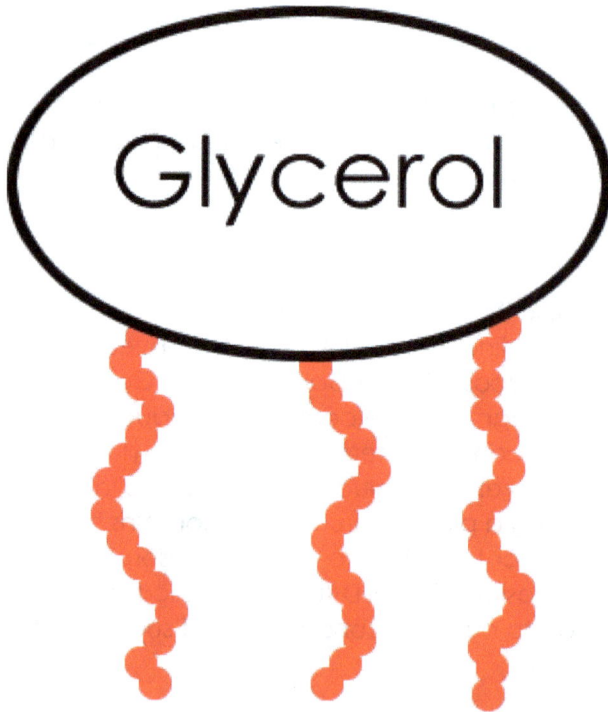

Figure 6.3
The structure of fat: glycerol with three fatty acids (triglyceride)

Fat is broken down by lipases (fat enzymes) from the pancreas into the form which can be absorbed across the gastrointestinal barrier. This form is glycerol (with one chain of fat connected called a monoglyceride) or free fatty acids (not attached to glycerol).

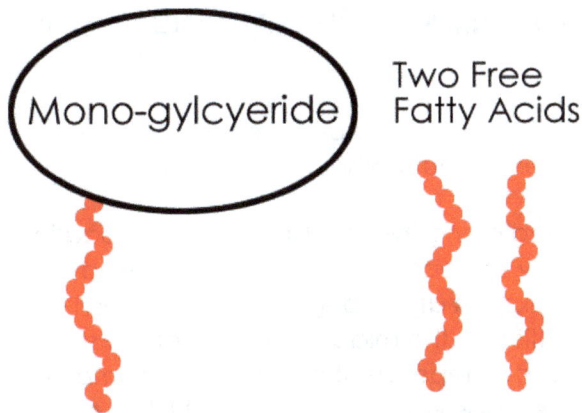

Mono-gylcyeride

Two Free Fatty Acids

Figure 6.4 The two forms of fat that can be transported across the gastrointestinal barrier are monoglycerides (glycerol with one fatty acid) and free fatty acids.

Unlike proteins and carbohydrates, fats do not require special enzymes secreted by the intestinal cell to be completely digested for transport. Monoglycerides and free fatty acids are directly transported by the lymphatic system and are dumped directly into the blood. Because of this, fats are more easily tolerated by a compromised system and produce fewer symptoms even if the cell villi are damaged. Fat soluble vitamins (Vitamins A, D, E and K) are transported at the same time as fats.

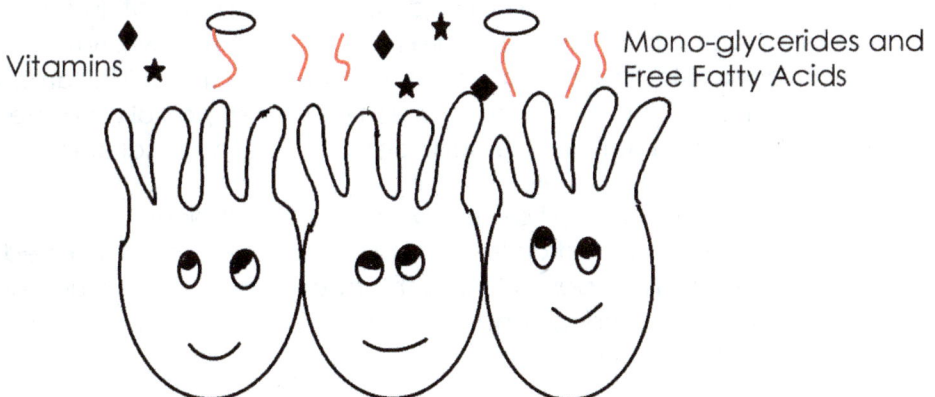

Vitamins

Mono-glycerides and Free Fatty Acids

Figure 6.5 Fat-soluble vitamins (A, D, K and E) are absorbed with monoglycerides and free fatty acids across the gastrointestinal barrier

6.4 MICRONUTRIENTS: MINERALS AND VITAMINS

Micronutrients are small enough to be taken through the gastrointestinal barrier without further breakdown.

Minerals are absorbed along the small intestine. The location depends on the body's needs. For example, if your body is low in calcium, it can be taken in at the beginning of the small intestine (duodenum) in addition to the middle and end of the small intestine. This transport is dependent on vitamin D. Some calcium can even be passively absorbed in the large intestine or colon. Other minerals such as iron, phosphorous, copper, and zinc are absorbed along the small intestine once they are released from the food you have eaten.

An important note about supplementing zinc is that excesses of zinc minerals can result in a copper deficiency. I recommend using the two together, typically in a 10:1 Zinc: Copper ratio. [4]

Vitamin absorption also occurs throughout the course of the intestine. The complexity of this process is beyond the scope of this book, but I have included a reference from the journal of biochemistry if you are looking to delve more deeply into this. [5]

The intestinal cell will not and cannot transport protein and carbohydrate foods that are not fully broken down. But, if the gastrointestinal barrier is compromised and the cell is damaged or not connected to its adjacent cells, then partially digested foods can get into the body between the intestinal cells.

Intestinal cells must be tightly attached to their neighbor cells to maintain the gastrointestinal barrier and prevent undigested food from sneaking past and into the body, where the immune system will see it as foreign and begin to attack it. (This is the trigger for Inflammation.)

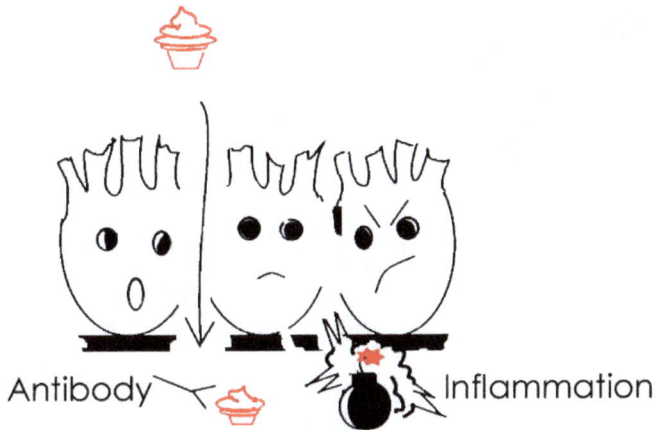

Figure 6.6 *Leaky-gut syndrome (LGS) results when intestinal cells are not tightly attached to each other. Undigested food can cross a damaged gastrointestinal barrier. The immune system then makes antibodies to protect you as it does not recognize the undigested food. This triggers INFLAMMATION and now you have become sensitized to this food.*

It there is not a tight cell-to-cell attachment, the gastrointestinal barrier is compromised. The result is a leaky gut (*hyperpermeability*). This compromise allows the immune system to be in direct contact with undigested food and leads to a myriad of health problems both in the digestive system and elsewhere.

Additionally, unhealthy intestinal cells are unable to produce the enzymes that do the final digestion of food. In this case, you do not need to have bacterial overgrowth for SIBO (small intestinal bacterial overgrowth) symptoms. When the intestinal cells are unhealthy, food can ferment in the presence of normal bacterial levels or irritate the intestine, resulting in symptoms of gassy bloating, diarrhea or constipation.

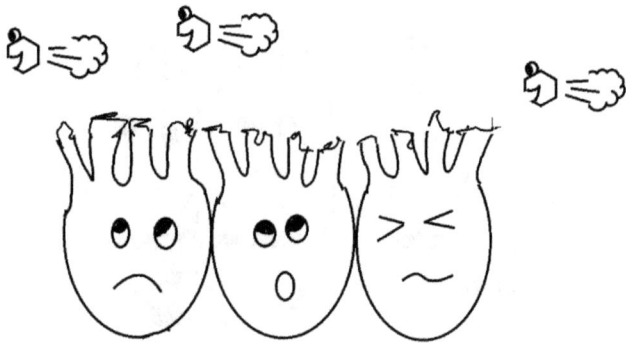

Bacteria produces gas from
food that sits in the intestine.

Figure 6.7 *Blunted Intestinal Cell Villi. When the gastrointestinal barrier cells are damaged, the fingerlike projections on the absorbing surface can be part of the damage. When this occurs, the cells are less likely to release the final enzymes for digestion. Food then sits in the intestine, serving as fuel for the bacteria and yeast which then produce gas. This occurs even with normal populations of bacteria and yeast.*

7 THE THREE PRIMARY REASONS FOR IBS/ SIBO

With these simple illustrations on nutrient transport, we've covered what I believe to be two of the primary causes of the symptoms of IBS and SIBO.

One is the health of the intestinal cell. What is especially important is the health of the brush borders that release the final enzymes to break down carbohydrates and proteins for transport into the body. Also important is the health of the tight junctions between the cells which create the gastrointestinal barrier.

The second cause of symptoms is an unbalanced microbiome (bacteria and other species). We now recognize that the microbiome, in addition to its protective functions in the intestine, also directly communicates with our innate immune system. This is an important component of whole-body health. [6]

The health of the intestinal cell and the health of its environment, including the microbiome, are critical and paramount to the healing of IBS/SIBO.

If the intestinal cell is not healthy, then unwanted bacteria and yeast species can settle in the small intestine and cause increased symptoms of IBS/SIBO. If the bacteria or yeast species settle in the large intestine, it results in Dysbiosis (microbial imbalance) of the Microbiome of the large intestine.

Bacteria and yeast live in our intestine. Some are beneficial to the microbiome, and some are not.

The third cause of IBS and SIBO includes deficiencies of pancreatic enzymes, gallbladder bile, and gastric HCL (acid).

In my experience, damage to the migrating motor complex (MMC) is secondary to the damage to the intestinal cell. For this reason, I do not consider this to be a primary cause of IBS or SIBO.

Food intolerance can be an additional source of inflammation and damage to the intestinal cell. This intolerance is a protective mechanism by the immune system and occurs because of a breakdown in the gastrointestinal barrier which allows the immune system under the intestinal cell to have a direct interface with the contents of digestion.

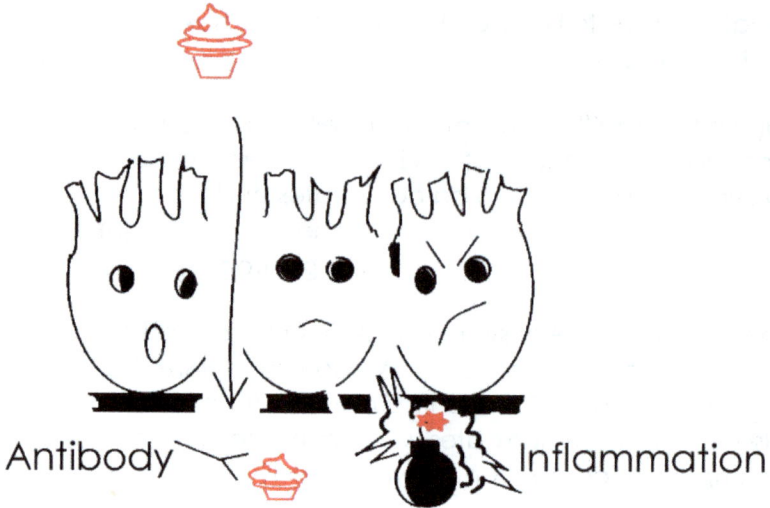

Figure 7.1 *Immune system and undigested food interface*

If undigested food gets between the cells and into the blood stream, the immune system reacts to protect you with inflammation. This is because these undigested foods trigger the immune system which goes into an inflammatory response to the food as if it is a foreign entity that you need to be protected from. Since the immune system only recognizes the smallest building blocks of food, it is natural that when it sees anything more complex, by default it sees it as a foreign invader and goes into an emergency response.

More about that in the Leaky Gut Chapter.

8 LGS AND THE GI BARRIER

The GI Barrier is paramount to your health.[7]

The idea of "leaky gut" has been evolving for some time now and functional medicine doctors have been using this as a basis for treatment of disease states for decades. As patients who suffer from the symptoms of IBS and SIBO begin to look for answers for the cause of their symptoms, they will surely come across the concept of leaky gut. If we want to be more medical in our terminology, we can refer to leaky gut as *gastrointestinal hyperpermeability*. (*Hyper* means increased, and *permeability* means ability to permeate or move through). You could also refer to it as a breakdown in the gastrointestinal barrier.

Anyone who has studied medicine and cellular histology in medical school will have studied the concept of cell adhesion. They will know that cell to cell adhesion is imperative to restrict movement of substances between the cells so that the cells get to choose what they will or will not transport. This is the way the intestinal cells become a selective membrane (allowing only what they want to pass through).

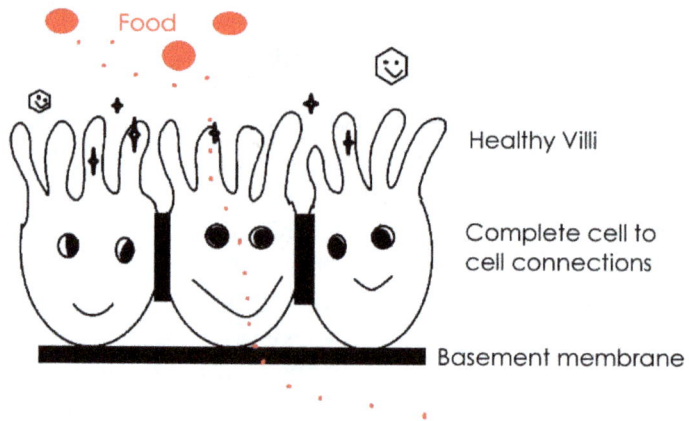

Figure 8.1 *A Healthy gastrointestinal barrier is comprised of a strong basement membrane that holds the cells in place, complete cell to cell connections and healthy intestinal cell villi that release the final enzymes for digestion. These elements result in selective absorption of completely digested foods.*

The following are lecture notes from Yale University cell biology class.

"Tight junctions perform a critical function besides cell adhesion. They restrict the diffusion of molecules between neighboring cells (*paracellular*). Tight junctions regulate the passage of ions and small metabolites, and the tightness of the diffusion barrier varies with the location of the epithelium: brain (tight), intestine (looser). In fact, the electrical resistance of some epithelia can differ by over 1000-fold.

Tight junctions are networks of strands that encircle the cell and interact with similar strands on neighboring cells to form a seal around the cells. Tight junctions are linked intracellularly to actin filaments that stabilize the junctions."[8]

The importance of the gastrointestinal barrier and the Microbiome are just beginning to have greater acceptance in the larger medical community. So, if you are up against someone who has a science background but is still operating from the old way of thinking, they may disregard the importance of Leaky Gut and its role in IBS/SIBO and perhaps even IBD symptoms.

This delay of acceptance occurs because emerging information challenges the model of current thinking. Often, the acceptance of an emerging medical concept becomes expedited when a drug treatment is developed to fix the problem and marketing is promoted around the concept. The drug representatives teach doctors about their product and advertising teaches the patients.

An example of this is with the drug Xifaxan or Rifaximin. This drug has been around for a long time and was previously approved for one specific disease; the treatment of hepatic encephalopathy. Prior to growing conventional interest in the importance of the microbiome, this was its only FDA-approved use. With the emerging information on the importance of the microbiome, Xifaxan is now FDA-approved for use in IBS-D.

Now that SIBO can be diagnosed with a breath test, it is on the medical radar. A diagnosis and prescription treatment are available in the form of Xifaxan; however, it is not FDA approved for use in SIBO. I have had the need to prescribe Xifaxan only a handful of times since its approval as a treatment and have seen unimpressive results relative to the use of nutrient and herbal based medicines.

The causes of gastrointestinal barrier damage are many and can accumulate over the years. They include the use of oral antibiotics and steroids, chronic cortisol release in stress, food reactions, pancreatic and HCL deficiency, dietary protein and carbohydrate irritations, infections, blood sugar issues, inflammatory antibodies, food allergies, environmental toxicity, early exposure to foods, internal toxicity and hormonal changes.

8.1 WE ARE BORN WITH A LEAKY GUT

We are born with a leaky gut. When we are born, the small intestine has not completely developed, and the cells have not fully joined up to create a solid, selective tube.

The bones in the skull and the alveoli of the lungs continue to develop after birth (the lungs will develop additional alveoli until 14 years of age). Likewise, the intestine and the immune system surrounding the intestine continue to develop for the first 2 years of life.

During the first two years of life, while the gastrointestinal barrier is completing development, it is an incredibly important time for dietary consideration. Because the gastrointestinal barrier is not fully developed, there is a direct interface between food and the immune system. The ability to develop intolerance can start here in the form of Immunoglobulin G (IgG) reactions, or delayed hypersensitivity. Delayed hypersensitivity is a reaction that can occur anytime in a five-day window after exposure to the food in question. Please be aware that I am not talking here about Immunoglobulin E (IgE) antibody reactions, also called immediate hypersensitivity reactions. Immediate reactions are the classic allergy path and occur within minutes of exposure, they follow the standard pattern of allergy that includes symptoms of congestion, breathing difficulty, rash formation and even anaphylaxis. These IgE reactions have been observed to decrease in early life with small amount of food exposures.

In terms of immune system development, 80% of the immune globulin (antibody) secreting cells of the body are positioned around the tube of the digestive track. Antibodies are what the immune system uses to protect us from infection. The immune system surrounding the intestines is called Gastrointestinal Associated Lymphoid Tissue or GALT. The cells of the intestine and the GALT pass information back and forth. Together they develop to become a strong, protective system that recognizes what to protect you from (for example, infection) and what not to (for example, food).

This healthy development of a strong gastrointestinal barrier is very much influenced by dietary exposures, antibiotic exposures, clean food, infections and stress-free system development.

This is the reason that a slow and regulated food introduction to an infant is so important.

If a baby under two years old with a developing immune and digestive system is exposed to a food that is an immune-system trigger too early, the immune system naturally will go into protective mode.

This means the dendritic cells of the immune system will react to the food as if it is a foreign protein. The dendritic cells (antigen presenting cell) will then "present" this problem to the B and T cells in the GALT. The T cells initiate an inflammation reaction, calling more cells and fluid into the region, which produces swelling and inflammation. The B cells develop specific antibodies to what the body believes is an invasion.

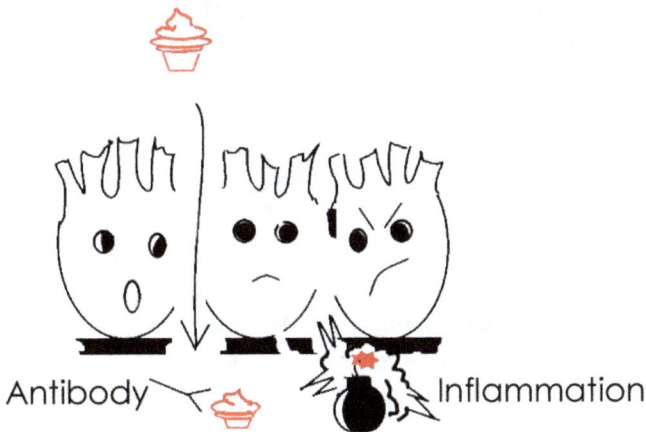

Figure 8.2 *Developing cells are forming their cell to cell connections and the immune system underneath the cells is also developing. The immune system is learning what to be on the alert for and can develop sensitivities to early food introduction.*

41

Now the body is sensitized. The immune system has developed an intolerance to the specific food.

The next time your baby's body sees that food, it will be prepared to attack, and it will give you a clear signal that it does not like it. This can be in the form of symptoms like colic, cramping, gas or reflux, and vomiting. In fact, I don't know if I believe that babies should be treated with acid blockers for reflux. What if babies don't get reflux but are really rejecting food, they are not ready for? They have no other way to tell us but to vomit or cramp up with colic. If we block their rejection response, then we're not solving the problem, but masking it. Before using acid blockers in babies, I recommend removing classing trigger foods from their diet and their mom's diet if she is nursing.

Over time, there can even be distant symptoms linked to foods as the immune system loses its vitality. This is because so much of the immune system focus is occupied by protecting the body from foods in the digestive system.

A baby whose immune system is weakened by food intolerances can have ongoing exacerbations of tonsillitis, otitis media (ear infections), breathing problems (asthma and congestion) and rashes (eczema).

I have lost track over the years of how many infants have come to my practice with parents beside themselves when their child was picking up one infection after the next and using course after course of antibiotic treatment. Once we found the offending food or in some cases GI overgrowth of yeast or bacteria and removed the problem, the baby's immune system could regain its strength and the chronic tonsillitis, ear aches, rashes and respiratory problems resolved.

Each time I see a new patient in my practice, during their intake I ask about a childhood history of tummy aches, chronic ear infections, placement of ear tubes, tonsillitis (apart from strep throat related), asthma and eczema. What I'm really asking is, did this problem start in childhood and has it been operating in the background of what we are witnessing as the current symptom picture?

This early antibody development against foods is also likely the cause for finding many IgG antibodies registering very high for some infants and children (and even some adults). In these cases, the gastrointestinal barrier never had the chance to fully develop. For these people, there has been a lifelong interface between the contents of the intestines and the immune system, causing a myriad of symptoms.

When I see a panel of IgG antibodies that shows reaction to all foods, I suspect that the problem began in infancy. Since you cannot eliminate all foods, we remove the most triggering foods as we go through the process of symptom recovery. It works beautifully.

> Here's a case of an 18-month-old boy with recurring infections which required repeat hospitalizations and many rounds of antibiotics. As soon as he recovered from one infection, he would pick up another ear infection or fever or tonsil infection or bronchitis. His mom was at her wits' end, and the doctors had advised her that they may run out of effective treatments for her son if he became resistant to the antibiotics they were using. The next plan was to remove the tonsils (enlarged due to constant immune challenges) and to place tubes in the ears to mechanically drain inflammatory fluids.
>
> His mom brought him to see me for an alternative course of action. We checked his blood for IgG antibodies and found them elevated to cow dairy, gluten and whole eggs. I explained to his mom that this constant immune insult by the foods he was eating could be behind all the infections, and if we remove the foods for a while, we'll know for sure. For 18-month-old children, this is so much easier to do because the diet can be managed more easily and there are so many more options for dairy and gluten and egg free foods available now. It may not be a surprise to learn that once the foods were eliminated, there were no more serious infections. He would pick up a cold virus like most kids and his immune system would take care of it in a couple of days. I asked the mom to keep him off the IgG foods for two years. Following that, she successfully re-introduced the foods to his then-stronger immune system and a less reactive digestive system. He is

now ten years old and continues to thrive without food restriction.

The following section describes my program for introducing food that I provide for my parents.

8.2 FOOD INTRODUCTION FOR INFANTS

Prior to 6 months, mother's milk, from a mom's healthy diet, provides infants with most of the nutrition they need. Some nursing moms need to take foods out of their own diets if their baby's system does not like them. If you are not nursing or need to supplement nursing, then a hypoallergenic formula is recommended. A rice or goat-based formula is preferred.

Introduction of trigger foods during early life may increase your child's chances of developing antibodies against foods which may manifest as dermatitis, colic, gassiness, constipation, reflux, chronic tonsillitis, chronic ear infections, severe teething episodes, chronic colds, flu, coughs, immune weakness, irritability or behavioral changes.

This occurs because the digestive tract and immune system are too immature to handle complex foods. When the time comes, introduce foods with these precautions in mind: The starred foods (*) have a higher ability to cause irritations and are introduced later.

Introduce only one food at a time and only when the child is well.

Do not try a new food sooner than every 5 days (weekly is easier to track).

Pay careful attention to your child's reactions to the new foods for 1-5 days after the introduction.

Reactions include colic, reflux, irritability, hyperactivity, unusual moodiness, skin rashes, blotchy cheeks, runny nose, congestion, or changes in bowel movements. Keeping a diary helps.

Please choose organic foods. Glyphosate (Round-up pesticide) residue has been found in many items, including infant foods.[9]

6 months	9 months	12 months	15 months	18 months
Mother's milk or hypoallergenic formula	Mother's milk or hypoallergenic formula	Mother's milk or hypoallergenic formula	Optional mother's milk from here on	
Banana	Papaya	Spinach, kale	Cauliflower	Pineapple*
Apples	Strawberries *	Chard	Tomato*	Orange *
Pear	Blackberries	Broccoli	Mushrooms	Peppers*
Peach	Green bean	Onion, garlic	Cabbage	Corn*
Plum	Nectarine	Potato*	Buckwheat	Wheat*
Blueberries (frozen for teething)	Raisins Peas squash	Parsnips Asparagus celery	Other nut butters (no peanut)	Corn flour* Sesame butter* Sesame oil*
Cherries (smash)	Zucchini	Oatmeal	Rye	Peanut*
Grapes (smash)	Sweet potato	Brown rice	Honey	Corn oil*
Yam	Millet	Barley	Barley malt	Eggs*
Carrots	Quinoa	Soy (tofu, milk) *	Egg yolk*	Beef*
Beets	Amaranth	Almond butter*	Lamb (no fat)	Pork*
	Basmati rice, peas	Hazelnut butter* Soy oil*	Fish (no shellfish)	Cow milk*
	Legumes (not soy)	Maple syrup poultry	Yogurt*	Cow cheese*
	Cold pressed oils	Miso, kelp, yeast	Chicken, turkey	
	Blackstrap molasses	Goat/sheep milk		

* starred foods have the highest potential to cause symptoms

8.3 LGS Functionally Defined

While the topic of LGS in infants may not seem relevant to you, exploring the developing digestive system in infants is a wonderful way to understand what leaky gut is like in an older body. I'm repeating myself here, but I want to really highlight this point as it serves as the center of the theory that has become my treatment protocol. For some infants, the digestive and immune systems get irritated by early exposure to foods like gluten or dairy or by infection and antibiotic use and never properly form. In these cases, the gastrointestinal barrier never develops to become the highly selective, transport membrane that we require.

You will see in the chapters on the anatomy of the digestive tract that the intestine is a tube which is continuous with the outside of the body and that food is not really "in" our body until it has been transported across the wall of the intestinal tube.

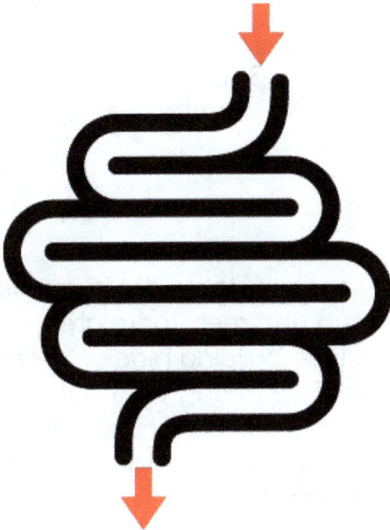

Figure 8.3 The Intestine is outside of the body!

The food we eat is not sterile. It normally contains bacteria, viruses, and yeasts. It is very important that the bacteria, viruses and yeasts or other infectious products move through the tube and exit our body in the stool. For this to happen, we must have very tight connections between the intestinal cell so that the intestine becomes a selective membrane, allowing *only* what the cells choose to transport through them and into the body. This is the gastrointestinal barrier. The intact barrier selects food building blocks for transport into the body and does not select bacteria. Here is the picture again of the components that comprise a health Gastrointestinal Barrier.

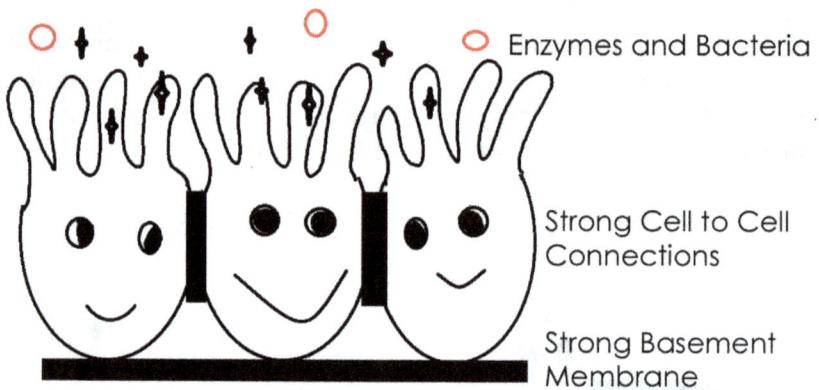

Enzymes and Bacteria

Strong Cell to Cell Connections

Strong Basement Membrane

Figure 8.4 *The selective GI Barrier*

In a healthy digestive tube, food is broken down into its smallest building blocks by stomach acid and enzymes. There are receptors on the intestinal villi for all the building blocks of food. In some cases, certain particles can diffuse through without receptors, once they are broken down into their smallest form. Receptors will grab the food building blocks and transport them selectively through the cell to the body.

Receptor

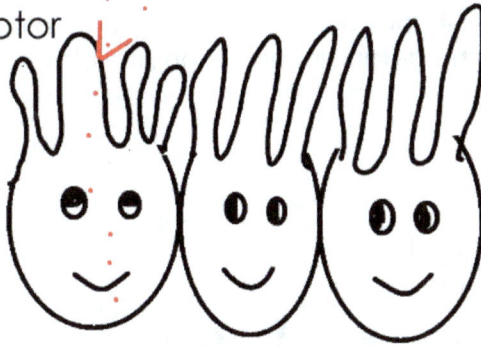

Figure 8.5 *Selective transport by receptors allows to cell to choose only completely broken-down food.*

Once in the body, they are taken for processing (usually to the liver).

With a leaky digestive tube, the gastrointestinal barrier is compromised. There are spaces between the intestinal cells which enable larger food pieces to leak between the cells into the blood stream. These spaces exist either because the system was never able to fully develop, or because of one of the irritating factors that promotes leaky gut was present. When these larger food pieces leak into the body, this is an <u>emergency</u> for the immune system.

The immune system recognizes the building blocks of food and allows them to pass into the body. But if food complexes that are larger than the single building blocks pass between the intestinal cells of a damaged gastrointestinal barrier and enter the body, the immune system sees them as foreign particles. The immune system thinks that the body is being attacked by what it interprets as foreign particles and goes on high alert.

The immune system sees anything that it does not recognize as food as a threat and will mount an inflammatory attack when it detects any unrecognized entity. This is not difficult for the immune system to do, since the selective transport into the body requires only the recognition of twenty amino acid and three carbohydrate building blocks, plus the vitamins and minerals. Therefore, the list of what it needs to recognize as normal is much shorter than the default list of foreign particles.

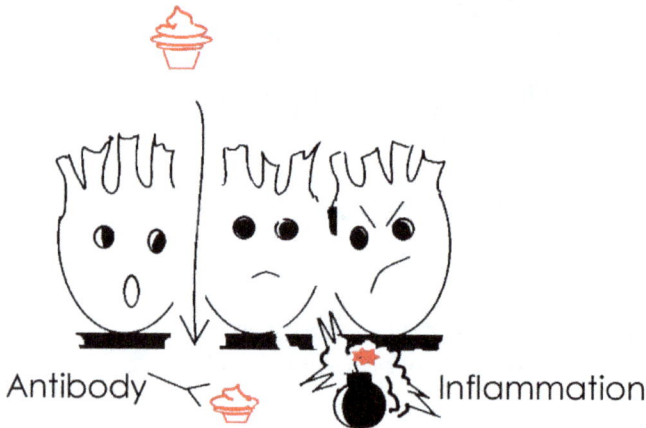

Figure 8.6: *The damaged GI barrier*

Once the immune system detects the threat of a foreign entity, it signals the release of inflammatory chemicals and antibodies. If the immune system is constantly exposed to these foods that are leaking, the inflammation becomes constant and gastrointestinal symptoms such as pain, gas, diarrhea and constipation result. Constant inflammation leads to more gastrointestinal barrier damage. Unless the food is removed, this becomes a vicious cycle of inflammation and increasing food intolerances.

The antibodies that are commonly associated with this problem are delayed hypersensitivity antibodies (IgG). These are different from classic IgE food allergies, in which the symptoms are immediate and can be life threatening. IgE antibody reactions involve the histamine pathways and cause difficulty breathing, throat closing, rashes and swelling. For these reactions, people typically carry an epi-pen. We can call IgG types of reactions "food intolerances" to distinguish them from IgE food allergies.

IBS/SIBO associated antibodies are in the class of delayed reactions and are typically mediated by IgG antibodies. Since these antibodies are delayed, the symptoms from them can occur anywhere up to five days after exposure to the food. There may be several foods producing antibody reactions. This can make isolating the food or foods that are a problem quite difficult. Fortunately, there are now several labs that test for these IgG antibodies to foods. These labs are functional medicine labs that offer specialized IgG testing. The IgG antibody is tested from a blood sample.

I have compared the results of IgG antibodies in the same blood sample run from conventional labs. When I do this, invariably almost every food I run comes out positive. We call this a false positive. It's no wonder to me that most gastroenterologists claim that everyone has IgG antibodies to any foods they have eaten, since most gastroenterologists use conventional labs. There is a different method of sensitivity and detection used when IgG panels are run through a functional lab which reduces the rate of false positive responses substantially, but not entirely.

Unfortunately, after more than two decades of helping so many patients resolve their IBS/SIBO symptoms with the results of their IgG testing, most insurance companies are still considering this test "investigational". However, I believe that it is worth your effort to do the test. The IgG reactions are not permanent but are a guide to eliminate irritations while the digestive system regains its strength.

Once your body begins to produce antibodies to foods, each time you ingest that food, the inflammatory reaction will be initiated either right away or for up to five days later.

You could compare this to the protection you get from your immune system when it encounters a cold virus. Once your body sees a unique virus, antibodies are produced and the next time you are exposed to that same virus, you are ready to attack it and stop it before symptoms start. The reason you catch another cold in the future is because there are hundreds of different cold viruses and they are constantly mutating. The difference between making antibodies to a virus and making antibodies to foods of course is that you want the protection from the virus, you don't want it from foods.

After detecting your IgG reactions, the real work begins. For the most part, the foods that can be linked to IBS/SIBO symptoms are cow dairy, gluten, wheat, eggs, sugar, yeasts, peanuts, corn, citrus, and soy. For some people, there are some other less common foods that are a problem.

If you're wondering why people with a leaky gut are not sick all the time from bacteria getting into their bodies through the intestine, the answer for is *size*. The size of an amino acid building block is 0.8 nanometers. The size of a very small bacteria such as Mycoplasma is 150-250 nanometers. [10] So, you can see that something as small as a couple of amino acids can sneak through a leaky gut, but even the smallest bacteria is too big.

8.4 WHAT CAUSES LGS

There are a variety of reasons for the damage to the gastrointestinal barrier in IBS/SIBO patients, but by far the most common are food intolerances, early food introduction to an immature system, stress during development, oral antibiotic or steroid use, and toxic exposures. This includes eating highly processed, manipulated, chemically exposed foods.

A controlled infant food introduction is extremely important for initially developing a healthy digestive and immune system so that a strong gastrointestinal barrier can form.

The main problematic foods for adults are cow dairy, gluten, sugar, yeast, soy, and eggs. For children, add to this list citrus, peanut, and corn.

We can control the food we select to eat, and we can choose minimal exposure to processed and chemically-laden foods.

We can use lifesaving treatments like antibiotics and steroids judiciously, and when they are needed, we can ensure that we replace and repair damage from their side effects.

I have seen many patients recover from chronic IBS/SIBO symptoms by employing treatment based on these concepts. As a result, I have a lot of faith in these steps to recovery. I trust that once we determine food irritations, replace digestive deficiencies, balance the microbiome and heal the cells of the intestine and stomach, we can have symptom-free digestion without extensive dietary restrictions.

I think the hardest part of the process is the food elimination. I like to assure my patients that this will usually be a temporary removal of the irritant until the system heals, regenerates and can tolerate this food again.

Our bodies can be irritated by infections, overwhelmed by toxic exposures and irritated by improperly-digested foods. The response of the body, though, is always the same. The body responds with inflammation. Sometimes, the actual irritant may no longer even be present, but it has acted as a trigger and now the body is locked into an inflammatory process. We call this "Chronic Inflammatory Response Syndrome." This takes us into a whole different area of treatment which generally requires immunotherapy or treatments of underlying factors to stop the reaction.

9 FAST TRACK TO GAS AND BLOATING RECOVERY

~GI Janel One– for IBS/SIBO gas, bloating & pain

For those of you ready to fast track, I recommend that you skip ahead to the instructions for dosing of GI Janel One. For a significant percentage of the population, the initial steps used to identify your food triggers and support your digestion may not even be necessary to repair and resolve your gas and bloating. This includes:

- People who have gas and bloating that is trapped and uncomfortably distending the abdomen
- Those with gas and bloating who pass copious amounts of gas
- The painful symptom of trapped gas that causes cramping pain in episodes or is ongoing.

The IBS/SIBO cases that respond well to the GI Janel fast track are those patients who notice that regardless of what they eat, their gassy symptoms occur day after day. Everything seems to "feed" the gas and bloating. In fact, the only reprise from symptoms is just to not put anything in their mouth. I also include patients in the fast tract category who will have their gas and bloating symptoms daily like clockwork with or without food. If you're fast tracking, I do recommend that the use of GI Janel One is accompanied by a soft food diet for the most impact. You can also add in digestive support in the form of GI Janel Digest formulas. You can read about these further in the GI Janel Family chapter.

> Here's an example of a fast-track patient in my practice. A 43-year-old woman came in with symptoms that have been ongoing for 13 years. They started following a Cesarean section delivery. For the past 10 years, she had been taking antibiotics daily for her acne which worsened her GI symptoms. She reported extreme gas pain and excessive gas that caused her abdomen to be distended. She reported burping (eructation) and flatulence all day long. She typically moved her bowels once a week, so her

diagnosis was IBS-C with suspected SIBO or SIFO. A colonoscopy revealed nothing abnormal, but her constipation was worse following the procedure. She had tried the Fodmap diet, but this did not change her symptoms. We did an IgG panel which came back with some very mild reactions to dairy and bakers' yeast. She then did an elimination and challenge of these foods and none of her GI symptoms changed during either the elimination or the challenge.

I began her on GI Janel One and GI Janel AM/BM and had her ramp them up gradually. When she returned in four weeks she reported that her gas and bloating were much improved. She still was burping quite a bit but noticed that this decreased when she ate more slowly. Her bowels were moving daily and were formed but thin. As a side note, she told me that her acne cleared up when she was off dairy, so she planned on keeping that out of her diet. I had her keep her GI Janel One dose at one tablespoon and added in my soluble fiber formula to increase the stool size. When she returned in four weeks, she reported that she was no longer gassy daily but did have some episodes of gassiness each week. I suspected that she was mixed SIBO/SIFO (bacterial and fungal overgrowth in the small intestine) and gave her a two-week dose of Diflucan to kill any yeast overgrowth, which eliminated these episodes. Obviously, she was very happy that after thirteen years of symptoms, we were able to clear them up in a matter of a few months.

I would like to highlight something important about this case. I ordered only one test for this patient. I ordered IgG food reaction testing which, while not helpful for her GI symptoms, was helpful to improve her acne. I did not test her for SIBO as it was obvious that she was having SIBO symptoms. It then it became a process of listening to her recovery to infer that she was SIBO and SIFO positive. It is not that I don't want to do the SIBO test, but I tend to reserve it for when the treatment protocol is not progressing as I would expect.

10 ANATOMY OF IBS / SIBO

Now we're going to examine the anatomy of the digestive system. If you understand the structure of your digestive system, it will be much easier to understand how it functions and to understand the underlying causes of your IBS/SIBO symptoms.

10.1 THE DIGESTIVE TUBE

The digestive process consists of digestion, absorption, and elimination.

Digestion is the breakdown of the food we eat into micro-molecular building blocks.

Absorption is the movement of these building blocks from the intestinal tube into the body.

Elimination is the exit of the waste from what we eat and leaves the digestive tract as stool. This includes waste and fiber that cannot be absorbed.

The digestive tract is essentially a tube made of cells that runs through the center of the body. It is open system because it is open on one end as your mouth and the other as your anus. Throughout its course, the tube changes shape, function and size, but it remains a continuous tube.

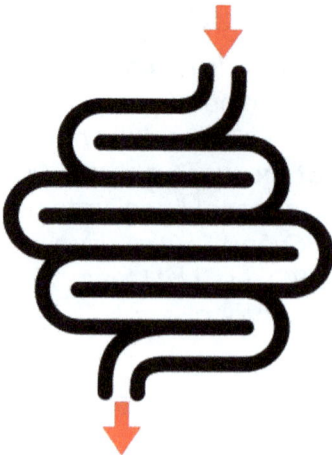

Figure 10.1 Digestive tube

Even though food is in the middle of the tube running through your body, the food is not actually in the body. You may not have thought about it this way before, but when food is in the digestive tube, which is continuous with the outside of your body via the mouth and anus, *it is outside your body*. As you can see in the picture below, food only enters your body after it crosses through the intestinal cell and into the blood stream. It is then carried for processing, usually to the liver.

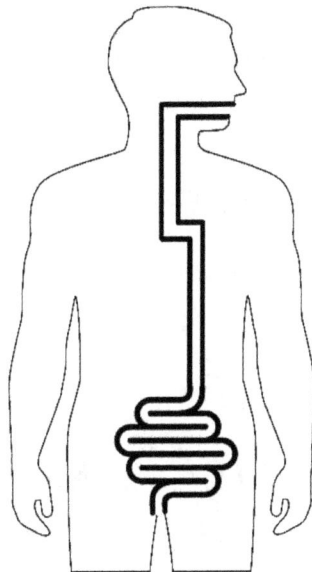

Figure 10.2 *The intestinal contents are outside of your body*

The concept of food being outside of our bodies when it is in the digestive tube is important and is critical for understanding why IBS and SIBO occur. Please keep this concept in the forefront of your mind.

10.2 KEY POINTS

- Food in the digestive tube is on the *outside* of your body (Figure 10.2).

- Food is not sterile, and the environment that we live in is not sterile. Sterile means that something has been cleaned of all bacteria and other infectious agents like viruses and yeasts.

- The GI barrier must be healthy and intact (Figure 10.3).

When you eat, you are consuming bacteria, yeasts, viruses, and sometimes parasites. You want these to exit in your stool (staying outside of you) and not to cross over the intestinal cells into the body.

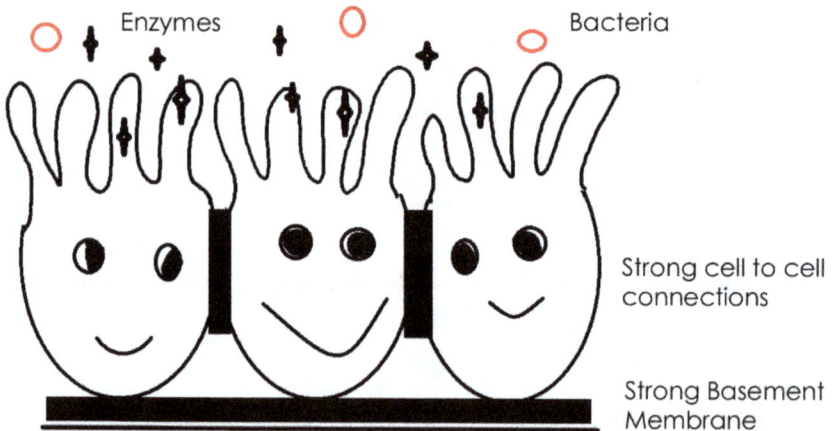

Figure 10.3 *A healthy GI barrier separates the undigested food in the intestine from the immune system under the basement membrane.*

10.3 INFECTION AND INFLAMMATION

When you go to the hospital for a surgery, the equipment is sterilized and handled very carefully to keep it free of anything that may cause an infection in your body. If there are bacteria on the surgical equipment, they can be introduced into your body. Once the incision is closed with sutures, those bacteria are trapped inside of you and can begin to multiply. When this happens, you can become critically ill. When you have bacteria multiplying and spreading in your body tissues, you are septic.

Whenever you see -itis at the end of word describing a body part, it suggests inflammation and often infection in that body part. For example, gastritis is inflammation in the stomach lining which may or may not have an infection present. Inflammation means that your immune system is trying to protect you by enlisting cells, fluids and inflammatory chemicals to the area of damage or irritation. When inflammation antibodies are attacking tissues of the body, it is called an auto-immune disease process.

As another example, diverticulitis is inflammation in the diverticula or pockets that balloon off the colon or large intestine.

DIVERTICULOSIS and DIVERTICULITIS

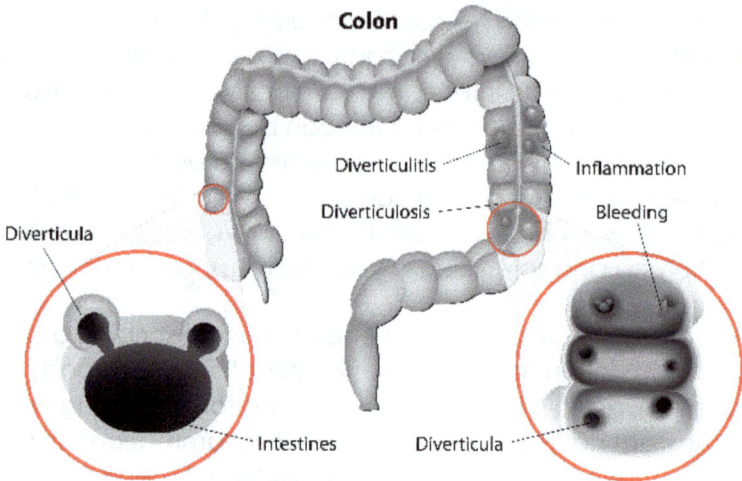

Colon

Diverticulitis

Inflammation

Diverticulosis

Bleeding

Diverticula

Intestines

Diverticula

Figure 10.4 Colonic diverticula are balloons that can form on the surface of the colon or large intestine. These may or may not be infected.

Diverticulosis is the presence of those balloons. Diverticulitis occurs when the balloons are inflamed and infected with trapped bacteria. This is a medical emergency and requires immediate attention or the balloons may rupture sending infection into your abdominal cavity.

Another example of bacterial sepsis in the body happens during an appendicitis rupture. The appendix is a little wormlike appendage that hangs off the first part of the large intestine. It can become infected with bacteria and become inflamed and painful. If the appendix ruptures, these bacteria are released into your body and make you septic. This is an emergency and requires urgent care.

The point that I'm trying to make here is that we can get critically sick when bacteria get into our bodies. But, when we eat, we are continually swallowing live yeasts and bacteria. It is very important that those stay on the outside (in the tube) and move through and out of the system with the waste. We do not want them to cross over through the gastrointestinal barrier and get into the body.

Our bodies are covered with skin to protect us from infection getting in. Bacteria, viruses and yeast are everywhere in our environment. When you have a cut or open sore, it must be cared for until it heals over, otherwise you risk infection setting in. We bandage cuts, scrapes or ulcers and apply topical antibiotics to keep bacteria out until the skin has healed over and is protective again.

When we eat, we take food which has microscopic yeasts and bacteria on it and put it all right into our mouths!

The transport of food from the digestive tube into the body must be highly selective (we call this the *gastrointestinal barrier*) so that only food and <u>not</u> bacteria or yeast are transported across the gastrointestinal barrier and into the body. We want the bacteria and yeast to be killed as they move through us. This is accomplished by the acid in the stomach or enzymes released along the way. We want most of these microbes to exit us as waste.

For the permanent resolution of IBS/SIBO, it is imperative that only food which has been completely digested (broken down) is absorbed (transported by the intestinal cells) and that we have a fully functional, healthy gastrointestinal barrier. A healthy digestive system can move bacteria and yeast along and out of us so that it cannot overgrow in the small or the large intestine. If you only kill the bacteria of SIBO and do not repair the gastrointestinal barrier or the Migrating Motor Complex (MMC), bacterial overgrowth can return and often does.

11 DIGESTIVE ANATOMY

11.1 THE NERVOUS SYSTEM

The "Brain" of the digestive tract is called the Enteric Nervous System (ENS). The ENS is unique. It can operate independently from the rest of the nervous system. This has earned the ENS the title of "The Second Brain" since even when cut off from input from the brain, it continues to function.

The ENS is one of three branches of the *autonomic* (think *automatic*) nervous systems. These are systems that operate without conscious involvement. For example, when you want to pick up a book you are consciously moving your arm to complete this task. When you are eating, you can consciously chew your food, but once you have swallowed it the rest of the digestive process is carried out without your conscious input (until the very end).

Stress is a principal factor in IBS symptoms and is the reason for the prescription of depression or anxiety medications to mitigate symptoms. Stress impacts the Enteric Nervous System because the ENS is most like the parasympathetic branch of the autonomic nervous system.

The parasympathetic nervous system (PNS) oversees rest and regeneration. PNS is responsible for the slow, gentle peristalsis or muscle movements that are continuously moving food through your intestines in wave like motions. They are so gentle and rhythmic that you cannot even feel them. This movement is what your doctor is listening for when they do your abdominal exam. We determine movement by listening for bowel sounds per minute. An IBS/SIBO system sounds too quiet in some areas and erratically noisy in other areas where the peristalsis is ineffective

The PNS acts in the opposite manner to the third branch of the autonomic nervous system called the Sympathetic (Stress) nervous system (SNS), which is responsible for the adrenal panic and the fright and flight response.

When your body is in sympathetic mode, it is preparing to fight or flee. The SNS Sympathetic nervous system prepares the body for emergency situations while parasympathetic nervous system maintains conserving functions when the body is at rest.

In SNS activation, the priority is not digestion as digestion is a conserving function. The blood supply is shunted to the muscles (for running away) and away from the digestive system. This reduces oxygen and nutrients to the digestive system and reduces effective peristalsis (muscle movement) in the intestines.

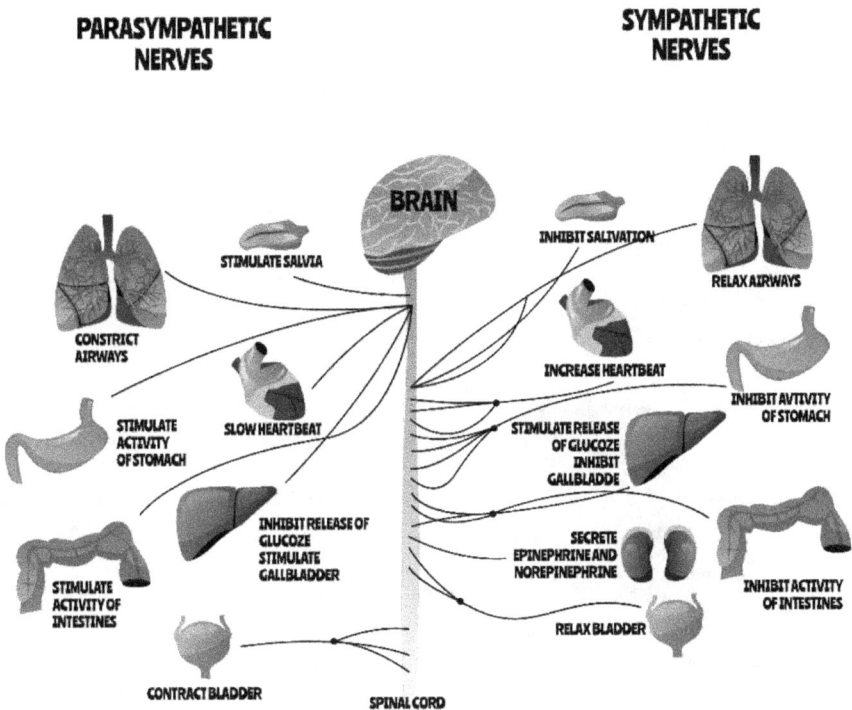

PARASYMPATHETIC NERVES　　　　　　　**SYMPATHETIC NERVES**

BRAIN

INHIBIT SALIVATION

STIMULATE SALVIA

RELAX AIRWAYS

CONSTRICT AIRWAYS

INCREASE HEARTBEAT

INHIBIT AVTIVITY OF STOMACH

STIMULATE ACTIVITY OF STOMACH　　SLOW HEARTBEAT

STIMULATE RELEASE OF GLUCOZE INHIBIT GALLBLADDE

INHIBIT RELEASE OF GLUCOZE STIMULATE GALLBLADDER

SECRETE EPINEPHRINE AND NOREPINEPHRINE

STIMULATE ACTIVITY OF INTESTINES

INHIBIT ACTIVITY OF INTESTINES

CONTRACT BLADDER　　　SPINAL CORD

RELAX BLADDER

Figure 11.1 *Sympathetic and parasympathetic supply to the digestive system. The system receives commands from the Parasympathetic (PNS/ENS) for gentle, rhythmic movement, rest and assimilation. The Sympathetic (SNS) can override the PNS under chronic stress and shift to commands of flight and fright. This decreases nutrient and blood supply. Overtime this can contribute to compromised health of the digestive system.*

When the body is under constant anxiety or panic, blood is shunted away from digestion and the digestive system. It then becomes compromised due to the decreased oxygen and nutrient delivery required to keep it strong and healthy. This is one of the ways that the intestines experience the damage to the gastrointestinal barrier that leads to IBS/SIBO symptoms.

It is interesting that over 90% of the body's serotonin (the neurotransmitter that increases with the use of SSRI medications) is not in the brain but in the ENS of the digestive tract. Drugs to increase serotonin or stimulate serotonin receptor sites in the ENS have been developed, but clinically offer little symptom relief for the IBS patient. [11] [12]

11.2 Mouth- Mechanical Digestion

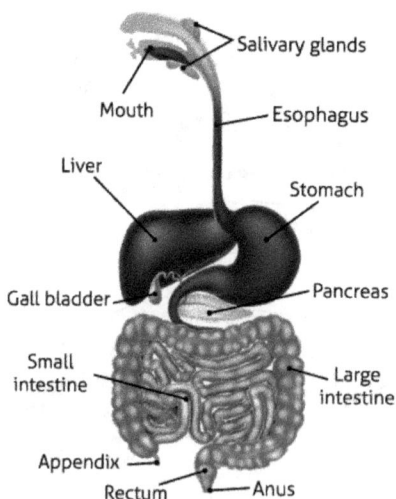

Figure 11.2 Digestive Anatomy

The digestive tube starts at the mouth, where the mechanical breakdown of food occurs during chewing or mastication. In the mouth, the saliva mixes with the food to form the food bolus which is swallowed.

Remember that digestion means breakdown.

The first digestive enzyme is called salivary amylase. It is released during chewing and starts to breakdown carbohydrates. The taste buds are in the fuzziness on your tongue (they look like little raised tires on their sides). These can send messages to the stomach and brain when components of food are detected chemically, so that the lower part of the digestive tube can prepare for what is coming.

Chewing your food well is so important because the only mechanical, crushing digestive process is in the mouth. After the mouth, the remainder of the digestive process is primarily chemical rather than mechanical. The more food is chewed, the more successful the chemical aspect of digestion will be. This is because chewing increases the surface area of the food, putting it in greater contact with the digestive enzymes along the rest of the tube.

11.3 ESOPHAGUS- TRANSPORT TO THE STOMACH

Once the food has been swallowed, it travels through the esophagus. The esophagus is the tube that connects the mouth to the stomach. After you swallow, the rest of digestion and the absorption of the food is completely unconscious and is under the control of the enteric branch of the autonomic (automatic) nervous system (ANS).

The smooth muscle that surrounds the digestive tube creates a slow, rhythmic movement called peristalsis. It is this gentle, wavelike motion that propels the food through the tube. The junction between the esophagus and the stomach is controlled by a one-way valve called the LES or lower esophageal sphincter.

This valve opens in a downward direction when it is healthy. No real digestion happens in the esophagus except for a little carbohydrate breakdown that was initiated by salivary amylase in the mouth.

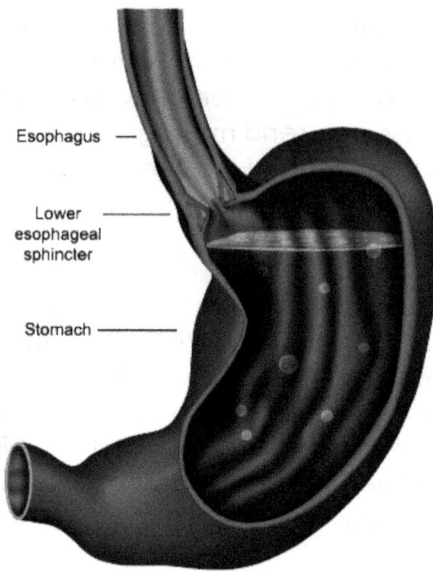

Esophagus —

Lower
esophageal
sphincter

Stomach ——

Figure 11.3 Esophagus to stomach

11.3.1 An aside on Heartburn

Reflux or heartburn occurs when the acid that is meant to be in the stomach moves through the LES valve upward into the esophagus. This may occur because the LES (lower esophageal sphincter) can no longer close properly and cannot keep the acid contained in the stomach. Reflux can also occur because the stomach has herniated up through the diaphragm.

Some risk factors for developing reflux include consuming meals that are too large, smoking and obesity. When the top part of the stomach herniates through the diaphragm, acid can more easily move into the esophagus. This is called a hiatal hernia. A hiatal hernia can be detected by an upper endoscopy or EGD (EGD stands for esophagogastroduodenoscopy, which refers to the esophagus, stomach, and duodenum). An EGD is a scope that allows your doctor to see the inside lining of the esophagus through to the first part of the small intestine.

The size of your empty stomach is the size of your clenched fist. It can obviously stretch substantially, but if it is continuously overstretched, it can become damaged in its structure and its physiology.

Long term use of pain medications called NSAIDs (Ibuprofen, Naproxen, Aleve, Advil, Aspirin) and alcohol will decrease and damage the protective layers inside the esophagus and the stomach causing or worsening heartburn symptoms, inflammation and ulcers.

The most common functional cause of heartburn is the inability of the LES to remain closed, followed by the inability of the valve separating the stomach from the small intestine to open properly (pyloric sphincter). Both valves are controlled by acid release.[13]

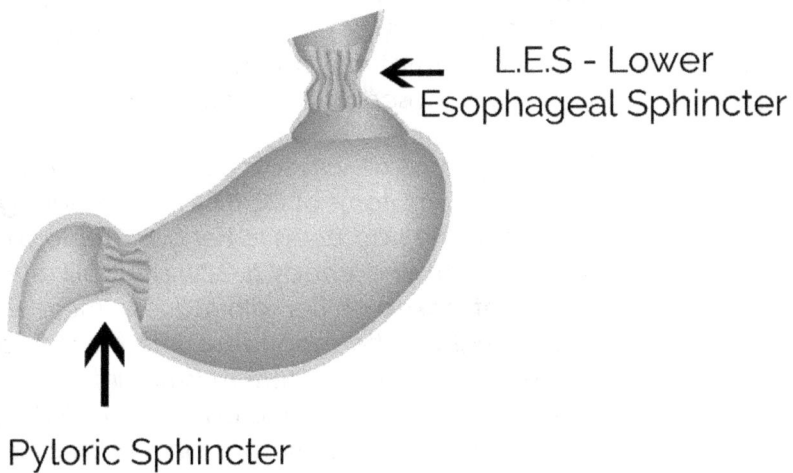

L.E.S - Lower Esophageal Sphincter

Pyloric Sphincter

Figure 11.4 *Reflux / GERD / Heartburn. Stomach acid signals the closing of the valve to keep stomach acid from moving up through the lower esophageal sphincter and into the esophagus. Stomach acid also controls the pyloric sphincter.*

The stomach itself is a very muscular bag with three layers of muscles running vertically, horizontally and diagonally.

The food enters the stomach and is churned around by these muscles. If the stomach cannot empty into the small intestine, the contents can move upward and cause heartburn symptoms. Nearly 90% of the patients that I treat for heartburn, regardless of the anatomy of the LES (damaged or functioning well), have resolution of their heartburn when we provide them with the signals that allow the valve from the stomach to the small intestine to open. This chemical signal seems to include the acid of the stomach itself. So, in many cases, providing the system with more acidity and digestive support during meals, rather than blocking acidity, improves reflux. This will not be the case in gastritis or esophagitis or H pylori infection. For these conditions, acid blockers are required while the system is strengthened and repaired. [14] [15]

There are many examples where simply increasing the acidity during digestion and/or increasing the pancreatic enzymes have resolved reflux. Here is one such example that not only demonstrated relief of symptoms but also repair of the digestion system confirmed by endoscopy and biopsy results.

> In 2015, a long term, 62-year-old patient reported severe and worsening symptoms of GERD (gastroesophageal reflux disease). She had been to her gastroenterologist and was given an endoscopy (EGD). Her EGD revealed raw tissue that looked on fire with redness. There were raw patches throughout the esophagus, into the stomach and into the first part of the duodenum (small intestine). She tested negative for H pylori and cancer. The EGD gave her a diagnosis of gastritis, metaplasia, peptic stricture (abnormal narrowing), esophagitis, erosion and Barrett's esophagitis, which is a pre-cancerous condition. I'll tell you, just looking at the lining of her upper digestive system made if obvious that she was in a lot of pain.
>
> My plan was to keep her on her acid blocking drugs while we determined if any food irritants were causing this inflammation, and to provide high doses of soothing and regenerating supplement support. This is an example of a very tender and sensitive system that would not be a good candidate for acid increase until it is fully repaired. I put her on a prescription of sucralfate (protective) and hyoscyamine (for esophageal spasms). She continued her

PPI (proton pump inhibitor), and we added an H2 blocker for breakthrough symptoms. From the natural pharmacy, I had her start GI Jan-aloe which is a concentrated mucopolysaccharide for healing tissue and immune system stimulation. I also requested that she brew and drink calendula flower tea daily, as this increases cell division and repair of the inflamed tissues. [16] Her symptoms were debilitating and would breakthrough even on the medications, so she kept on hand baking soda, Deglycyrrhizinated licorice chews, liquid antacids and Pepto-Bismol.

After 10 months of this treatment, her symptoms improved to the point where we could cut her prescriptions back to the PPI along with the healing formulas. She noticed that her symptoms improved off grains and was eating a paleo type diet. As her system became stronger, it was time to begin to support her digestion with a very mild digestive enzyme which she tolerated well. I also added in GI Janel One for cellular repair.

In 2018, it was time to repeat the EGD and see how the tissue inflammation was. Two polyps were removed and biopsied benign. Apart from some minor irritation at the LES where the stomach and esophagus meet, there was no gastritis, no metaplasia, no peptic stricture, no erosion and the Barrett's esophagitis was gone.

11.4 STOMACH – ACIDIC DIGESTION

The stomach is a muscular bag. It churns and mixes up the food you've chewed and swallowed and exposes it to an acidic pH. The enzyme called pepsin is also released in the stomach. At the correct pH, pepsin will begin protein breakdown.

Your stomach is roughly the size of your clenched fist. It can expand to accommodate the volume of approximately 4 liters or 1 gallon. There are receptors that fire when the stomach wall is stretched, which tell the brain that the stomach is full. If the signals of fullness are ignored or if the stomach is constantly being overstretched, you may lose the ability to receive these signals.

During digestion, stomach acid can get as low as a pH of one. This is the pH level of battery acid.

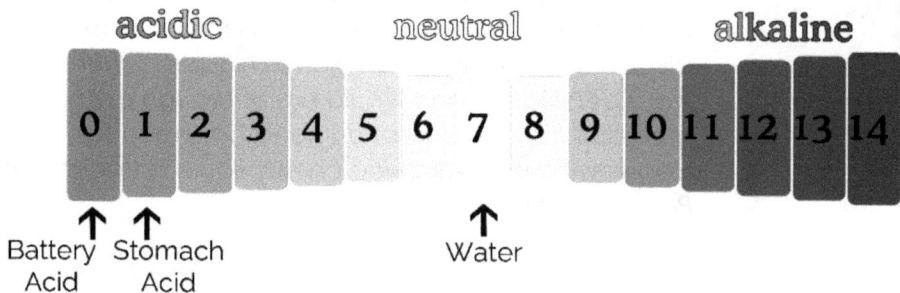

Figure 11.5 *Stomach acid is very acidic (low pH)*

There are many reasons that this acid level is important.

First, the enzymes that begin the breakdown of proteins in your food work best in this acidic environment.

Second, the acidity protects you by killing the bacteria and other pathogens that we ingest with our food. Remember our food is not sterile. We need many protective features throughout the tract to ensure that we don't get sick from the critters that come in with the food we eat (see chapter on leaky gut syndrome and the gastrointestinal barrier).

Thirdly, the acidity in the stomach is needed to begin the process of vitamin B12 and mineral absorption. Studies show that people on long term acid blockers can get more infections, are more prone to osteoporosis (weakened bones) and can have lower levels of B12 which results in fatigue. [17] [18] [19] [20] [21]

Because the pH is so strong, we need to have a lot of protection lining the stomach so that a hole doesn't burn right through it (this is an ulcer). The protection is in the form of a thick mucus layer which stops the acid from burning the stomach wall. When this protective mucous layer is worn down due to overuse of alcohol, NSAIDs or stress, the stomach acid can cause damage and erosion to the stomach and esophagus. and acid blockers will need to be used while it is healing.

Surface Mucous Cell
Covers the inside of the stomach

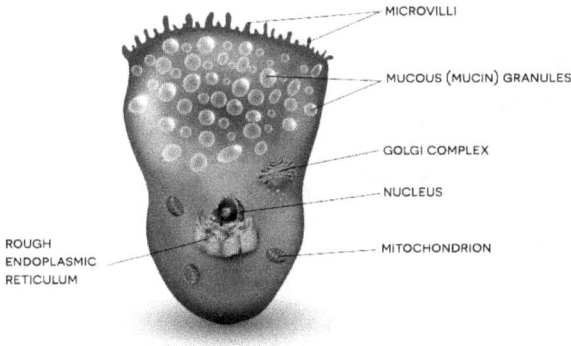

- MICROVILLI
- MUCOUS (MUCIN) GRANULES
- GOLGI COMPLEX
- NUCLEUS
- MITOCHONDRION
- ROUGH ENDOPLASMIC RETICULUM

Figure 11.6 *Protective mucus lines the stomach*

11.5 SMALL INTESTINE – ALKALINE DIGESTION AND ABSORPTION

pH of the gastrointestinal tract

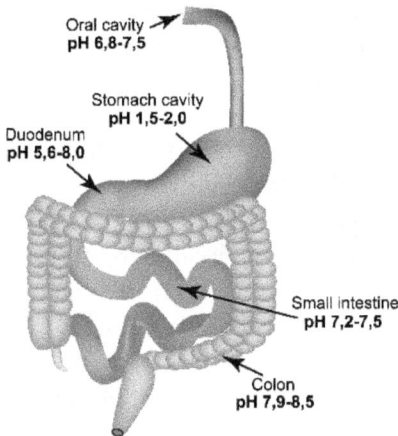

Oral cavity
pH 6,8-7,5

Stomach cavity
pH 1,5-2,0

Duodenum
pH 5,6-8,0

Small intestine
pH 7,2-7,5

Colon
pH 7,9-8,5

The small intestine is where most of the digestion (breakdown) is completed. When the food moves along the small intestine, it should be completely broken down so it can be properly absorbed.

Absorption occurs when the food is microscopically transported through the wall of the small intestine and into the body. The small intestine is approximately 25 feet long and one-half inch in diameter, consisting of folds and more folded folds. The smallest fold of this system can be called the "brush border" because it looks like the bristles on a brush.

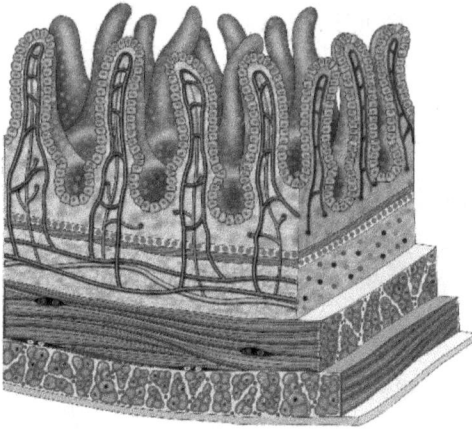

Figure 11.7 Brush Border
Absorption means
transport into the body

These layers of folding provide a huge surface area for transport. The surface area of the small intestine is so large that if it were spread out flat, it would cover close to half a tennis court in area.

The first part of the small intestine is called the duodenum. The primary function of the duodenum is to continue the digestion of food that began in the stomach. The pancreas and gall bladder secrete enzymes and bile into tubes that dump into the small intestine. These enzymes mix with the food travelling through and break it down. The pH of the small intestine is alkaline rather than acidic (like the stomach). The enzymes from the pancreas work better in this environment.

The food travels through the three parts of the small intestine: the duodenum, jejunum and ileum. The food is pushed along by rhythmic peristalsis or contractions of the smooth muscle wall. These contractions are controlled by the parasympathetic nervous system which instructs the smooth muscle wall of the intestine. The food mixes more and more with the enzymes that are breaking it down. When the food is broken down small enough, it can be transported through the intestinal wall and into the body.

Once in the body, the food nutrients are taken to the liver for use in the body. You can appreciate now how important it is to chew your foods very well so that the food can be better exposed to the enzymes for breakdown and absorption.

Remember that food is still outside of the body *until* it is taken across the intestinal cell and into the blood.

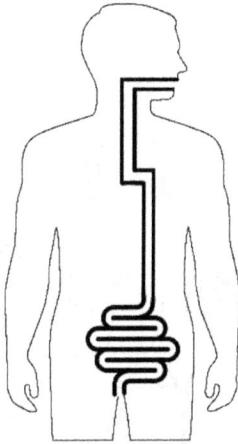

Figure 11.8 *The digestive system is continuous with the outside of the body.*

Protein building blocks are call amino acids, and carbohydrate building blocks are called monosaccharides. These are transported to the liver through the blood vessels along with water soluble micronutrients (vitamins and minerals) which have been extracted from the food. Once at the liver, they are used to build, repair, provide fuel and maintain the health of all the body tissues.

Since understanding this absorption process is critical for getting at the functional cause of IBS/SIBO, we looked at it in much greater detail in the Leaky Gut chapter previously.

11.5.1 Carbohydrate Digestion

Carbohydrates are starches made of maltose chains, lactose and sucrose. Their final breakdown occurs at the level of the small intestinal cell, just before they are transported across the gastrointestinal barrier. This digestion is not accomplished by enzymes that come from the pancreas, but by enzymes that are released from cells in the brush border of the small intestine.

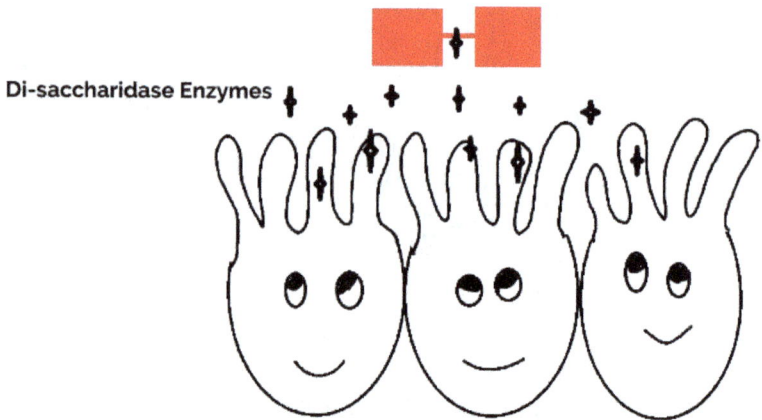

Figure 11.9 Brush border enzymes break di-saccharides into mono-saccharides for absorption into the body

These enzymes are called *disaccharidase* because they break down two (di) sugars (saccharides) into mono (one) saccharide.

- Maltase disaccharidase splits maltose into two molecules of glucose
- Lactase disaccharidase splits lactose into a glucose and a galactose
- Sucrase disaccharidase splits sucrose into a glucose and a fructose.

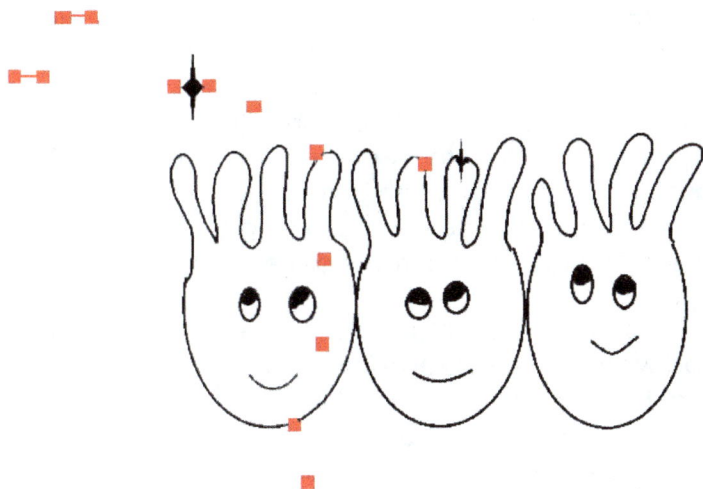

Figure 11.10 *Splitting a disaccharide for absorption into the body. Carbohydrates arrive at the gastrointestinal barrier as two, joined building blocks. The healthy intestinal cell releases enzymes to break them into single blocks. The single blocks can then be transported by the cell into the body. Anything larger than a single building block, cannot cross a healthy gastrointestinal barrier.*

Some people are carbohydrate intolerant – meaning they get symptoms of gas, bloating, diarrhea or possibly constipation from eating carbohydrates. The problem in these cases is that the health of the brush border is not adequate to sustain the cells which manufacture disaccharide breaking enzymes.

When carbohydrates cannot be broken into single building blocks, they cannot be transported across the gastrointestinal barrier. The carbohydrate will then sit in the intestine and ferment causing gas, bloating and diarrhea. If the bacteria living in the small intestine are imbalanced or polluted by backflow of bacteria from the large intestine (as in SIBO), this fermentation and irritation can occur very quickly.

So, even beyond SIBO, the poor digestion of carbohydrates is a result the health of the intestinal cell. If the cell is healthy and releasing these enzymes, the carbohydrates can break into single building blocks and can be transported into the body. Otherwise, they stagnate in the small intestine and *encourage* bacterial overgrowth by providing the bacteria with fuel!

After treatment for IBS/SIBO with GI Janel, the system will have been repaired and strengthened. The carbohydrate intolerance decreases or resolves. The brush border regenerates its ability to release the disaccharidases. Gas, bloating and diarrhea stop without needing to restrict carbohydrates in the diet.

Fructose and glucose are monosaccharides and are ready to be absorbed without further breakdown. Eating these monosaccharides can cause IBS/SIBO symptoms due to the state of the microbiome and SIBO or SIFO fermentation. You can easily prove to yourself if you have SIBO or SIFO by eating a monosaccharide exclusively and subsequently experiencing gas and bloating symptoms.

In SIBO there is a population of bacteria in the small intestine which should not be there. There can also be yeast in the small intestine (SIFO, or Small Intestinal Fungal Overgrowth). Any of these critters can ferment the food coming though and cause gassy symptoms. People who have symptoms regardless of the type of food they eat or drink are typically harboring imbalanced yeasts or bacteria in their intestines.

> *Here is an example from my practice of a patient who was having a clear carbohydrate intolerance with her other digestive symptoms. Three years ago, I met a delightful patient who had lived with 25 years with IBS/SIBO symptoms. She had most recently been on the FODMAP diet, which provided a little relief. Based on what we've just learned, you might already have an idea of what is going on for her. Even when eliminating easily fermentable carbohydrates, her symptoms were not relieved. This is because she was not releasing proper amounts of intestinal disaccharide enzymes. This problem may be in association with normal levels of bacterial and yeast species. Additionally, she may have overgrowth of yeast and bacterial in the small and in the large intestine.*

She reported bowel urgency, frequency, diarrhea, abdominal pain, trapped gas, bloating and a feeling of burning in her digestive system. We first ran a test to determine any delayed food reactions and removed those foods. She kept to a low fiber, soft food diet to give her digestion some rest. We completed a SIBO test which showed no excessive bacterial overgrowth. This means that the gas and bloating are either coming from yeast species overgrowing, a bacterium that was not tested on the SIBO panel, or from a lack of intestinal enzymes. I started her on a version of my Digest B formula and GI Janel One to help support the repair of the intestinal cell function and balance the microbiome.

Once she had completed the course of treatment, she was removed from the full dose to a maintenance dose of GI Janel One. We added in some soluble fiber as prebiotic support and kept her on regular use of Digest B at meals. We continued to desensitize her to the long list of trigger foods that she initially had. These included cow dairy products, whole eggs, soy, gluten and bakers' yeast. She has since reported resolution of all gastrointestinal symptoms for the past two years, regular daily bowel movements and only experiences diarrhea when exposed to her one remaining trigger food (gluten).

11.5.2 Fat Digestion

Fats are digested (broken down) in the small intestine by bile from the gallbladder, which emulsifies the fat, and by pancreatic lipase, which further breaks fat down. Fats are then absorbed through the intestinal wall by simple diffusion or by fatty acid transporter proteins in the small intestinal cell wall. [22]

Unlike proteins (amino acids) and carbohydrates (monosaccharides), fats are not transported through the blood vessels to the liver. Instead, fats move into the lymphatic channels and then are dumped into the main blood stream where they circulate through the body.

This is the reason that you need to be fasting for your cholesterol panel (primarily for the triglyceride part). If you are not fasting and have just eaten a fatty meal, your triglyceride numbers can be misleadingly elevated.

11.5.3 Protein Digestion

Proteins are digested by proteases, or protein breaking enzymes. Similar to carbohydrates, proteins (concentrated in foods like animal meat and legumes) are digested almost all the way to amino acid building blocks by the time they reach the brush border for absorption.

The proteins, however, are not completely digested at this point. They are not ready to cross the intestinal cell and get into the body. They are still in the form of little joined proteins called peptides. In order to complete the breakdown into free amino acids, they must be chopped up by special peptidases on the surface of the brush border cells of the small intestine.

Just as in the case of carbohydrate digestion, protein digestion requires a healthy small intestinal cell that can release the final digestive enzymes, liberating the building blocks into a form where they can enter the body.

11.5.4 Fermentation and Irritation

We have now seen a critical step in the understanding of IBS/SIBO. Both carbohydrate and protein digestion depend on the health of the intestinal cell. The cell must be healthy enough to release enzymes that will complete the breakdown of food into the smallest building blocks that can then cross the gastrointestinal barrier. These single building blocks can then be transported by the cell into the body. Anything more complex than a single building block cannot be absorbed.

Both proteins and carbohydrates rely on the health of the intestinal cells to complete digestion. Healthy intestinal cells provide the enzymes that complete the final step of the digestive process. The intestinal enzyme finishes the final breakdown (digestion) of the food into a form that can be absorbed (taken through the cell and into the body).

If there is a compromise in the health of the intestinal cells, these final steps are not available. This means that the carbohydrates which have not been fully broken down cannot cross the intestinal cells and enter the body. Instead, they stay in the digestive tube and ferment, causing gas and irritation.

The same can happen with proteins that are not fully broken down. These proteins cannot cross the intestinal cells until fully digested. They can stay in the digestive tube and irritate the intestine. This inability to complete protein and carbohydrate digestion is one of the main causes of gas symptoms, regardless of overgrowth. There are a few exceptions, but for the most part, all dietary carbohydrates and proteins can serve as substrates for microbial fermentation. [23]

Fermentation produces volatile fatty acids, lactic acid, carbon dioxide, hydrogen and methane gas. Hydrogen sulfide gas can also be produced, as we'll see in the chapter on sulfur intolerance.

Through the course of your GI Janel treatment, once the system is repaired and the cells regain their strength and ability to function, fermentable foods begin to be tolerated. Major diet restrictions of fermentable foods (FODMAP, low carb, paleo) will no longer be necessary. As a matter of fact, once symptoms have resolved off fermentable foods, I often ask my patients to add them back in very gradually so that they act as prebiotics and keep the microbiome strong. Too much all at once is a bad idea. It's better to use these foods as gentle medicine and gradually increase them, coaxing the beneficial microbiome to a healthy state.

Once the intestinal cells are healthy again, they can produce the enzymes to complete the final breakdown of protein and carbohydrates so that the food can be absorbed into the body, instead of acting as an irritant in the intestine.

Interestingly, because fats do not require a final digestive breakdown at the intestinal cell (they have been broken down by bile and pancreatic enzymes), fats are the least irritating of the three macromolecules for SIBO/IBS patients.

As we explored in the "leaky gut" chapter, if there is enough inflammation, irritation or damage from exposure to irritants, antibiotics, steroids, NSAIDS or high, constant stress, the connection between the intestinal cells will be damaged.

When the gastrointestinal barrier is damaged, incompletely digested proteins or carbohydrates can "leak" into the body where they can be perceived as foreign and trigger the immune system to upregulate and attack. The inflammation triggered by these "foreign molecules" can result in digestive symptoms like cramping abdominal pain, diarrhea and constipation. This can occur independently of any overgrowth in the small bowel.

The antibodies that attack the food form immune complexes. An immune complex is the foreign entity with an attacking antibody attached to it. These are found in the stool and in the blood. Those in the blood can also be responsible for distant symptoms elsewhere in the body as the inflammatory response is now in the circulation. (See my chapter on the importance of infant food introduction). Many patients notice that if they remove irritating foods from their diet, suddenly long-term acne or dermatitis clears up or they may have less pain, more energy or a clearer mind. Many patients begin to realize when working with these concepts that food is a powerful medicine.

11.5.5 Lactose Intolerance, an example of fermentation and irritation

If our food is incompletely or ineffectively broken down, it can irritate the digestive system. For example, with lactose intolerance, the enzyme (lactase), which breaks down the milk sugar lactose, is deficient. Lactose is a disaccharide made of galactose and glucose. The lactase enzyme is missing because it is not able to be produced and released from the small intestinal brush border cells.

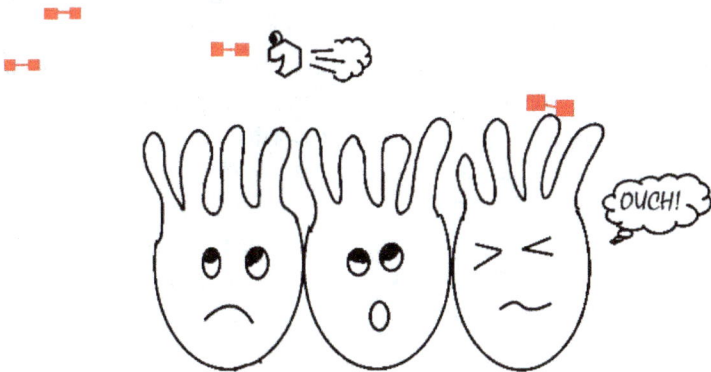

Figure 11.11 *Lactose intolerance: milk sugar (lactose) cannot be broken down into glucose and galactose because there is a deficiency of the enzyme Lactase. Glucose and galactose can cross the gastrointestinal barrier, but lactose cannot. As it sits in the intestine, it provides food for the bacteria which use it to make gas. It is also an irritant producing diarrhea to quickly rid your body of the irritation.*

When the lactose sits in the small intestine because it is unable to be broken into glucose and galactose as monosaccharides for transport into the body, it begins to ferment. This fermentation and irritation from the sugar results in abdominal pain, bloating, flatulence, nausea, and diarrhea beginning 30 minutes to 2 hours later. For some people, it is even more immediate.

If lactase deficiency is present at birth, it is termed congenital lactase deficiency. These babies must be fed lactose-free formula, or they can develop severe diarrhea, dehydration and weight loss.[24]

Many cultures do not have milk or dairy products as a regular part of their diets after infancy. These cultures obtain their calcium from other sources like green vegetables, legumes, nuts and seaweeds. Remember, adult cows don't drink milk, and yet they produce a calcium rich product.

If lactose intolerance occurs in adulthood, it is a result of lowered production of lactase enzyme in the brush border cells of the small intestine. If this phenomenon is due to damage of the cells by hidden infection, food intolerance, steroid use, stress, neurotransmitter dysregulation, neuropeptide dysregulation, immune dysregulation, early food introduction, or microbiome imbalance, then it can be categorized with the same gastrointestinal barrier damage that cause the other symptoms of leaky gut and IBS/SIBO. Likewise, if the proper healing steps are taken, the cells have the potential to regain their capacity to produce lactase so that dairy products can be tolerated without symptoms.

If the deficiency of the lactase enzyme is due to a deeper genetic or other cultural or congenital causes, then the body may never be able to processes milk sugar well.

11.6 PANCREAS- DIGESTIVE ENZYMES

In discussing the small intestine, we've already covered a lot of what the pancreas does because it is the pancreas that supplies the digestive enzymes to the small intestine.

The pancreas is made of two regions with distinct functions. The *exocrine pancreas* is the part that produces the digestive enzymes. The *endocrine pancreas* is the part that produces insulin and glucagon to regulate blood sugar levels. The exocrine pancreas releases its enzymes through a duct that flows directly into the small intestine. The endocrine pancreas releases its hormones into the blood where they circulate throughout the body.

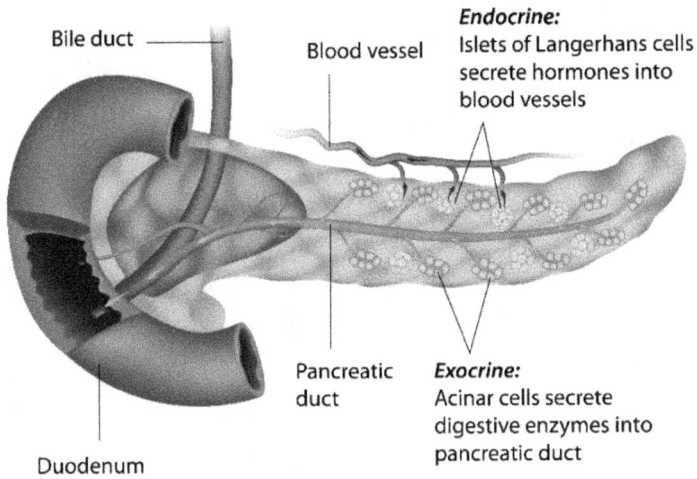

Bile duct

Blood vessel

Endocrine:
Islets of Langerhans cells
secrete hormones into
blood vessels

Pancreatic
duct

Exocrine:
Acinar cells secrete
digestive enzymes into
pancreatic duct

Duodenum

Figure 11.12 *The pancreas has two functions. The endocrine pancreas releases hormones into the blood. The exocrine pancreas releasees digestive enzymes into the small intestine*

Food is made of macronutrients and micronutrients. The enzymes from the pancreas break down macronutrients (fats, carbohydrates and proteins). (Micronutrients are minerals and vitamins.)

Macronutrients must be broken apart by enzymes into their building blocks to cross the GI Barrier	Micronutrients are ready to cross the GI Barrier
	Minerals: Potassium Magnesium Manganese Iron Phosphorous Copper Iron
Carbohydrates: Fiber, starch and sugards	
Proteins	Vitamins: Folate Thiamine (B1) Many other vitamins at lower levels of concentration.
Fats: Omega three fats, monunsaturated, polyunsaturated and minor saturated	

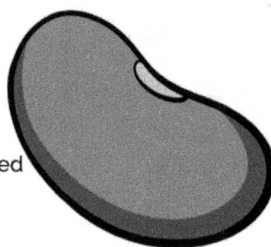

Pinto Bean

Typtophan: is actually a protein building block but is in it's single amino acid form and ready to cross the GI Barrier

Figure 11.13 Macro- and micro-nutrients in a legume (bean)

Here is an example from my practice of the impact of pancreatic digestive enzymes. A 24-year-old woman had been referred to me by a local physician. At her first visit, she told me about a three-year history of urgent and frequent diarrhea that she noticed after drinking coffee with cream. She cut out the coffee and cream, but her symptoms did not stop. Instead she began to have one week of frequent cramping, painful diarrhea all day followed by a week of normal bowel habits with no pain. This progressed to a point where she began to feel cramping pain daily, accompanied by a lower bowel pressure sensation that she needed to move her bowels but could not. She saw a gastroenterologist who did stool samples for parasites and calprotectin (inflammation). The results were negative. The gastroenterologist then put her on the FODMAP diet. The diet did not change her symptoms.

Two months before her visit with me, her symptoms flared up badly. She was having up to eight episodes of diarrhea daily and was managing her symptoms with Imodium and ibuprofen for the stomach pain. This was really taking its toll on her because she worked with the public and was having to excuse herself often. I put her on my GI Janel Digest B formula (pancreatic enzymes) with meals and some soothing digestion herbs while we waited for her food panel results.

When she returned four weeks later, she told me that if she misses taking her Digest B formula, she will have a rumbling in her stomach following meals and then will have diarrhea immediately. When she takes her GI Janel Digest B with her meals, she has no pain and no diarrhea. She said that this occurs regardless of what she eats. Since her food panel came back positive for antibodies to cow dairy, whole eggs, gluten and beef, I requested that she do an elimination and challenge of these foods and return with her findings.

She came back a few weeks later and told me that if she continues with her GI Janel Digest B formula, she can eat all the foods that came up in her panel without any symptoms of pain or diarrhea. At that point, she decided to just keep the GI Janel Digest B with her and take it with all meals, while limiting the foods in her panel. I love this example of simplicity. To resolve symptoms which she had for years, this young woman needed only to support her pancreatic release of digestive enzymes. I have been following her now at eight-week intervals for two years to ensure there is no re-occurrence of symptoms as we desensitize her to her IgG foods.

Pancreatic lipase breaks down fats. Pancreatic amylase breaks down carbohydrates and sugars and pancreatic proteases breakdown proteins. These all work best in an alkaline environment, which is why the small intestine the environment shifts from the acid environment of the stomach to a higher pH in the intestine. This pH change is accomplished by bicarbonate which is released from the cells lining the pancreatic ducts. In the stomach, the pH can be as low as 1, whereas in the first part of the small intestine (duodenum) the average pH is 6.6, and by the time the food reaches the end of the small intestine (ileum) the pH can be as alkaline as 7.5. [25]

11.7 Gall Bladder- Fat emulsifier

The gallbladder is a small sac that is located just under the liver. Bile is formed in the liver, and then moves into the gallbladder where it is stored in preparation for a fatty meal.

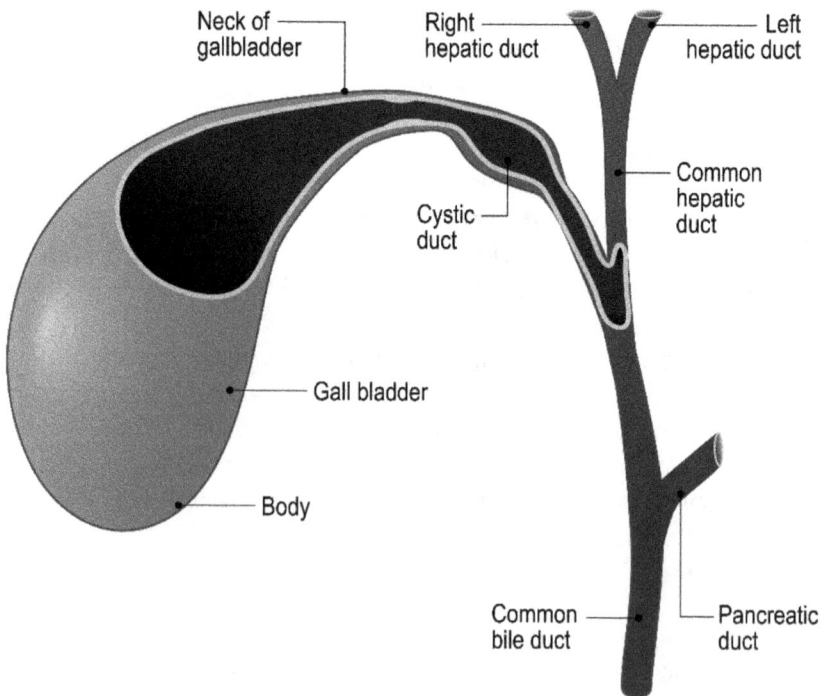

Figure 11.14 Gallbladder

Remember that bile is used to emulsify fats, which prepares them for breakdown by the pancreatic lipases so that they can be absorbed in the small intestine. When the gallbladder is full of bile, it is roughly the size of a pear. When fat is detected in the digestive system, a hormone called cholecystokinin pancreozymin is released, which causes the gallbladder to contract and squeeze the bile into the bile duct. The bile duct transports the bile to the small intestine. There, the bile contacts the fat and emulsifies it.

11.8 LARGE INTESTINE- ELECTROLYTE AND WATER TRANSPORT

In a healthy digestive system, by the time the food reaches the end of the 25-foot-long small intestine, all macromolecules have been completely digested (broken down) and absorbed into the body for use. What remains is a sloshy liquid. It is the responsibility of the large intestine (colon) to remove liquid and to balance electrolytes. Indigestible fiber is an important component of this liquid. The probiotic bacteria in the colon use this fiber as a food source and produce as a bi-product short chain fatty acids (SCFA). These SCFA are in turn used to maintain the health of the large intestine cells. It's a little ecosystem right inside of you.

Throughout the course of the digestive system, insoluble fiber is important for motility. Fiber is the only macronutrient that survives digestion. By escaping digestion breakdown, fiber maintains its structure, which gives something for the intestine to push against. Newton's third law states that for every action, there is an equal and opposite reaction. If there is nothing for the intestine to push against (fiber), then peristalsis (muscle contractions) that move substances through the intestines are compromised.

This can be a bit of a backfire for people with IBS/SIBO as introducing insoluble fiber too early can worsen symptoms. Eventually though, fiber will be an important part of your IBS/SIBO recovery. We just need to take it step by step and not overwhelm your body with things it cannot handle during repair and regeneration.

The large intestine or colon attaches to the end of the small intestine in the lower right corner of your abdomen. It then travels up the right side of your abdomen to just below the liver and ribs. At this point it takes a 90 degree turn and crosses the front of your body to the left side where it descends to the lower left corner of your abdomen.

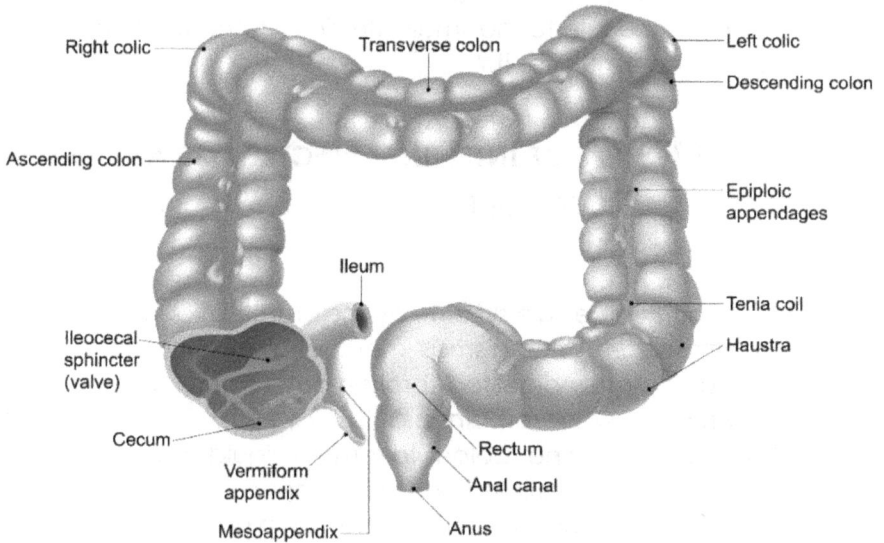

Figure 11.15 The colon (large intestine) starts at the end of the small intestine with a valve called the ileocecal valve. It then goes up the right side of the body as the ascending colon, across the body as the transverse colon and down the left side of the body as the descending colon.

The different areas of the digestive tube have different functions. The primary function of the large intestine or colon is water and electrolyte balance. The valve that separates the small from the large intestine is called the ileocecal valve or ileocecal sphincter. It is another one-way valve that prevents backflow from the large intestine (colon) into the small intestine.

The large intestine is about five feet long and is up to 2.5 inches in diameter.

The inside of the large intestine contains copious bacteria. We call these the beneficial bacteria, probiotics or the microbiome. It is important that these bacteria remain in the large intestine and have no contact with partially undigested food in the small intestine. If there is a backflow of the large intestine contents due to a faulty valve or motility (digestive movement) issues, then we can get symptoms. The backflow results in SIBO or SIFO and symptoms of gas, bloating and cramping. These symptoms occur because the bacteria can now ferment the partially digested food and cause gas to form.

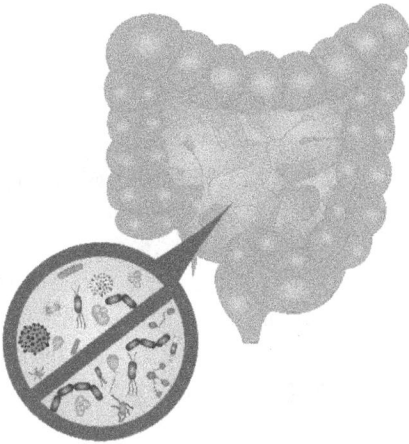

Figure 11.15 Backflow of bacteria from the large into the small intestine (SIBO)

By the time the food reaches the large intestine (also called the colon), it should have been broken down and transported into the body. In addition, about 80% of the water from the food has been absorbed into the body. The remainder of water is absorbed in the large intestine along with ions like sodium and chloride to make a solid stool. What remains is a sludgy waste that contains waste from the liver. The liver dumps waste into the digestive system along with the bile to get it out of the body. Also remaining in the system to form stool is the fiber that we cannot break down (insoluble fiber).

The large intestine or colon has four functions. It absorbs water and mineral ions, it ferments indigestible materials (fiber), it serves as storage for waste, and it houses a population of over 500 species of bacteria and some fungal and viral species.

When the fermentation of undigested fiber occurs in the large intestine, short chain fatty acids are formed, which serve as nutrients for the large intestine cells.

The bacteria in the colon also interact with the immune system and produce vitamins such as Vitamin K and biotin. We are now discovering that these bacteria can release hormones that can influence our moods. We are finding more about the importance of these bacteria all the time. Also produced in the large intestine and absorbed into the body are vitamin B1, B2, B6 and B12. [26] [27]

11.9 PROBIOTICS

Probiotics for the microbiome is currently a hot topic. There is much that we don't know about the microbiome, yet everyone is recommending probiotics, or so it seems. Not me. I don't want everyone to take probiotics. Many of these bacteria are transient species and they are going right through you and into the toilet. Many systems are not a healthy enough environment for the probiotics in a pill to seed and grow. Many will constipate and make an IBS/SIBO patient feel worse rather than better.

With a damaged MMC (migrating motor complex), as occurs frequently in SIBO, the organisms can become stuck in the small intestine and worsen symptoms of gas and bloating. It may be more effective to promote the growth of wanted species with a whole food diet. Studies show that the microbiome can change rapidly with a dietary change. [28]

Having said all of that, I will typically prescribe probiotics to patients with chronic or acute diarrhea symptoms. They can also be helpful for infants and children who are having digestive issues. Apart from these instances, I much prefer that my patients spend their resources on supplements that will repair their bodies and decrease their symptoms in an obvious manner.

The following are bacteria that are currently considered part of a healthy microbiome, according to Diagnostic Solutions GI Map testing. [29]

Bacteroides fragilis – Gram-negative species of the Bacteroidetes phylum. Immune-modulating normal gut species. Believed to be involved in microbial balance, barrier integrity, and neuroimmune health. High levels may result from reduced digestive capacity or constipation. Low levels may contribute to reduced anti-inflammatory activity in the intestine.

Bifidobacterium spp. – Gram-positive genus in the Actinobacteria phylum. Present in breast milk. Colonizes the human GI tract at birth. Common in probiotics. Thrives on a wide variety of prebiotic fibers. Low levels may result from low fiber intake or reduced mucosal health. High levels are more common in children than in adults.

Enterococcus spp. – Gram-positive genus of lactate-producing bacteria in the Firmicutes phylum. High levels may be due to reduced digestive capacity, constipation or small intestinal bacterial overgrowth. Low levels may indicate insufficiency of beneficial bacteria.

Escherichia spp. – Gram-negative genus in the Proteobacteria phylum. Normal gut flora. *Escherichia coli* (E. coli) is the primary species in this genus. Most E. coli are nonpathogenic. High levels may be indicative of increased intestinal inflammatory activity. Low levels may indicate reduced mucosal health and decreased protection against pathogenic E. coli.

Lactobacillus spp. – Gram-positive genus of lactate-producing bacteria in the Firmicutes phylum. Many strains used as probiotics. High levels may result from reduced digestive capacity or excessive intake of carbohydrates. Low levels may be due to low carbohydrate intake or high salt intake and may also indicate reduced mucosal health.

Clostridium spp. – Gram-positive genus in the Firmicutes phylum. The Clostridium genus is diverse and consists of both pathogens and normal commensals that perform a wide variety of functions (beneficial and potentially harmful). High levels may result from reduced digestive capacity or constipation. Low levels may be due to insufficient fiber intake.

Enterobacter spp. – Gram-negative genus in the Proteobacteria phylum. Closely related to *E. coli* (in the same taxonomic family). High levels may indicate increased intestinal inflammatory activity. Low levels may indicate reduced mucosal health.

11.10 SIGMOID COLON- TEMPORARY STORAGE

The sigmoid colon attaches to the end of the large intestine in the lower left corner of your abdomen. It essentially stores the formed stool until it exits the body.

The sigmoid colon is an "S" shape that stretches out into more of a linear tube if we squat. That's why there are products being produced to align the body in a squatting position during bowel movements. If the sigmoid colon is stretched, the stool can pass more easily through the straightened tube and there is less pressure built up our system. If there is less pressure needed to move the bowels, then we are less likely to form diverticular (balloons) in the large intestine wall. If there is less pressure, we are also less likely to develop hemorrhoids, which are engorged veins in the rectal area. Fecal matter can be stored in the sigmoid colon for 7 hours or longer.

11.10.1 Gastrocolic Reflex

The *gastrocolic reflex* is an important reflex triggered by food entering the first part of the small intestine. This reflex sends signals out to increase motility all the way down in the colon. The colon can then move the stool along so that a bowel movement can occur. Think about that: the system has a built-in clearing mechanism so that when functioning properly, you eat a meal and expel waste from a previous meal. In a completely healthy digestive system, it would be normal to have a bowel movement following each meal. This can still be seen in cultures which eat primarily whole foods (non-refined, non-processed, packaged foods), and it can also be observed with babies.

11.11 THE MUCOUS LAYER AND PROBIOTICS

The inner lining of the intestine is coated with a mucous layer. Two crucial functions of this lining are to protect you from being digested by enzymes and gastric acid (you are protein after all), and to provide a home for the probiotics. With no healthy mucous, there is no place for these important parts of digestion.

Mucous is made in the first part of the small intestine, called the duodenum. The bacterial density of the small intestine increases as food travels through it towards the colon. Some doctors prescribe plant-based treatments to support the mucous layer, like glycyrrhiza (licorice root), Althea (marshmallow root) or Ulmus (slippery elm bark). I have found that the concentrated Aloe mucopolysaccharide is also very effective for repair and maintenance of this important digestive mucous. [30]

Mucous is protective. When you have a cold, you produce mucous in your respiratory system. Why do you think this is? Well, the mucous is protective. The mucous is coating the virus and working with the immune system to eliminate the virus that you picked up. The body never does anything just to annoy you! It is trying its best to keep you healthy.

We use GI Jan-Aloe together with GI Janel One to repair the mucous layer of digestion and to repair the cells and cellular connections. By doing this, your body can regenerate the ability to produce and release final stage digestion enzymes from the brush border. Once the ecosystem has been repaired, the probiotics then have the environment that they need to flourish.

I cannot tell you how many hundreds of patients I have encountered over the years who have been taking probiotics only to find that when we do a stool test, they have low or very often NO GROWTH of those probiotics in their samples. I explain to them that the environment is not conducive to the growth of the probiotics they are taking, so those good little bacteria just shoot right on out.

Think about it this way. If a landscaper came to your home and planted trees without preparing the soil, you may have a lovely yard for a few weeks but before long the plants will be far from thriving and may even die. If the same landscaper prepares the soil with rich nutrients, then there is a much better probability of a long term, thriving garden.

If the soil (your intestinal tract) is properly prepared (by removing inflammatory foods, providing support to the digestive processes and nurturing and repairing the tissue and mucous layer) the probiotic species can then flourish and do their job to continue to keep you healthy.

You want probiotics because they are part of the ecosystem in your intestines that keep you healthy. They are involved in vitamin synthesis, natural antibiotic production, immune defense, digestion, detoxification of pro-carcinogens and they have a host of immune regulatory activities that are still being discovered.

But if the probiotics that you are taking end up in your toilet, that's a big waste of your time and money. Typically, I do not prescribe probiotics until the end of treatment except in some specific cases.

Some doctors recommend the avoidance of probiotics if you have SIBO. The premise here is to avoid more bacteria from seeding the small intestine. There is a risk of seeding the small intestine with the probiotics that are meant to live in the large intestine when the MMC (migrating motor complex) is damaged. For either reason, whether the probiotics get stuck in the small intestine or go right through you and into the toilet, I rarely recommend probiotics in the early cases of IBS or SIBO that I treat.

Avoiding the FOS (Fructooligo-saccharides) or other fibers that are added to some probiotics is also wise, as they can ferment and irritate in SIBO or SIFO and worsen gas and bloating.

Once the digestive system has been strengthened, probiotics are then fine to use to support further strengthening of digestion. If the weakened digestive system has been repaired, then the probiotics can potentially grow, and this will be helpful.

12 TRANSIT TIME

In a perfectly healthy digestive tract, there should be 2-3 meals moving through all the time. Transit time is the time that it takes a meal to move all the way through the digestive system and exit as waste.

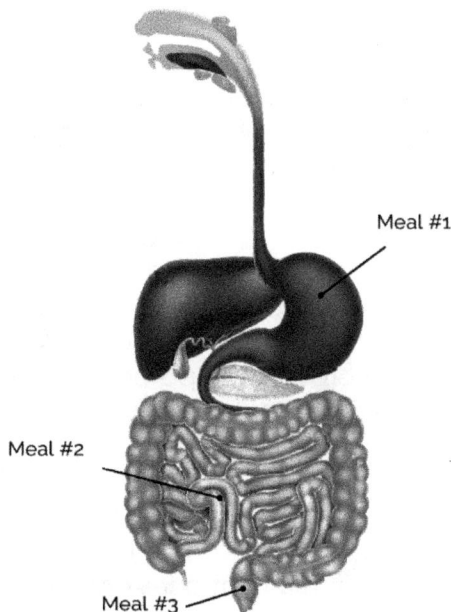

Meal #1

Meal #2

Meal #3

Figure 12.1 Transit time, a day of meals: digestion, absorption and elimination of waste.

First there is the meal that has just been eaten. Let's say it is dinner, which is getting churned in the stomach and moving into the small intestine.

The second meal is lunch from the same day, which should be completing digestion in the small intestine and moving through the valve into the beginning of the large intestine.

Thirdly, there is the meal that was eaten earlier at breakfast, which should be close to being fully processed and ready to exit the sigmoid colon through the rectum. The gastro-colic reflex helps this process by initiating contraction in the large intestine when the current meal moves from the stomach to the small intestine.

This is a rough overview, but with some give and take, it's how the system functions. If you're ever been told that it is not necessary to move your bowels at least once daily, that's just simply not true.

Most recent studies on transit time give an average of 40 hours for a meal to move through the body, which is more of a reflection on the current health of our systems and the quality of our diet.

You can easily test your transit time by eating something that will show up obviously on the other end. You can use beets or sesame seeds. When you see this food in your stool you will know how long it has taken for it to move through your digestive system.

If you've eaten three meals and have not moved your bowels, then there is an awful lot of waste sitting in your system. This stagnation creates irritation and heaviness in the colon. While the waste is stagnant in the bowel, there is also a potential to re-absorb back into your body the waste elements that the digestive system was trying to get rid of.

For example, the liver packages up excess hormones and sends them into the digestive system to exit the body. If there is stagnation in the colon, then the waste hormones can be re-absorbed through the entero-hepatic re-circulation. When your doctor is working on hormone balance in your body, they will need to address constipation issues as a part of this process. Also, a stagnant colon is the perfect environment for yeast to flourish. Yeast occurs normally in our intestine, but it can overgrow, allowing more disruptive yeast species to grow in a stagnant digestive system.

13 SYMPTOMS

Here is an example of a patient that I treated recently who came in with the perfect storm of all GI symptoms. Her digestive problems started in 2007 and persisted through to 2018 when she came in to see me.

She told me that in 2007 she had gone to the emergency room for rectal bleeding from a diverticulitis flare and was given antibiotics and IV pain medications. Since then she would have episodes of abdominal bloating that were very painful and would take months to resolve. She told me that in 2007, she went from size 14 to size 20 over the course of a few weeks. She was experiencing diarrhea with up to 12 bowel movements a day, followed by constipation with no bowel movement for up to 7 days. She was afraid to pass gas because she had experienced many episodes of bowel incontinence when attempting to pass gas. She had frequent episodes of left sided, upper GI cramping pain that she reported as severe. One of her unique symptoms was the inability to burp. She had pain associated with the pressure build up in her upper digestive system from this. She would drink soda to burp a little and this would relieve some of the gas pressure.

At her first visit in June of 2018, I started her on GI Janel Digest A with meals and GI Janel One at a 1/8 tsp dose. We did a patch test for foods and she came back positive for reactions to cow dairy, eggs, wheat, baker's yeast and soybean. She immediately eliminated all of these from her diet. When I saw her again in four weeks, she reported that her digestion was improving. She was able to burp to release gas after increasing her dose of GI Janel One to ½ tsp daily. I asked her to stay off the food irritants and continue her supplements.

When we met again in early October, she reported that all her symptoms were gone. She was having regular, daily bowel movements, her gas and bloating had been eliminated and the only GI pain that she had was in the lower abdomen with a diverticulitis flare. She knew her body so well that now she could tell when her diverticulitis was flaring due to the lower left abdominal location, whereas previously, when her entire abdomen was gassy and inflamed, it was hard to pinpoint what was going on.

We discussed a liquid diet and a chlorophyll enema treatment that she could start with diverticular flares. I advised her to go to urgent care if the enema was not resolving early episodes of diverticular pain. This simple treatment, which took four months, resolved over ten years of daily symptoms for this patient. Why is this? Because we removed the food irritations to put a stop to the chronic inflammation. We replaced the digestive deficiency, and we repaired the system with GI Janel One nutrients.

13.1 CONSTIPATION IS NOT A LAXATIVE DEFICIENCY

The title of this section is meant to be facetious. I'm trying to remind you that constipation is not normal, it is the body's way of telling you that it needs attention, as the system is not working well or is being irritated.

There can be rare circumstances where the nervous system or another system in the body is responsible for constipation. There also can be more serious GI issues such as a stricture or blockage; however, these are very rare. Ruling them out should be part of the diagnostic workup that you have. If constipation is not resolving or there are other symptoms that suggest there is something more serious going on, then imaging, such CT or MRI scans, should be done.

Chronic constipation is often a part of IBS symptoms. For some people, the constipation has been chronic for many years, and the other IBS symptoms like pain and gassiness start to add to the problem over time.

Pop quiz! If something is irritating your digestive tube and your body wants to get rid of it, what will your symptoms be?

Is your answer "diarrhea or vomiting"?

Trick question! Chronic irritants can also cause constipation, especially when the irritants are things like yeasts that have flourished in a weakened digestive system. Yeasts love to grow in a warm, dark, moist, stagnant environment. Yeast is anaerobic (it grows without oxygen). As it feeds on the sugars and carbohydrates that you eat, it buds and grows and releases gas and alcohol. As the host of this yeast overgrowth, you will have symptoms of gassiness, bloating and constipation, and for some people there may be episodes of diarrhea. We are finding that in SIBO, bacteria can do the same thing and decrease motility.

In a healthy, well-functioning system, your food will digest and move through your body in 12 –24 hours. You can easily test your "transit time" by ingesting something obvious and checking for it in your stool. Food like beets or sesame seeds work well. Remember digestion consists of three processes: breakdown of food, absorption (transport from the digestive tube into the body) and elimination (bowel movement of waste).

The symptoms of chronic constipation include: straining, hard stools that look like balls or rabbit pellets, a feeling of incomplete evacuation or going longer than 24 hours without a bowel movement.

Constipation can also occur as a secondary symptom to other conditions. It can be a side effect of a medication or can be secondary to diet, behavioral, metabolic, endocrine, neurologic or structural problems such as a stricture, cancer, anal fissure or proctitis (inflammation of the anus or lining of the rectum).

The prevalence of constipation ranges from 2-28% of the population, and accounts for 5.7 million physician visits per year. Constipation is considered more alarming if it is accompanied by bleeding, acute weight loss, obstructive symptoms or prolapse (falling out of place). [31]

The American College of Gastroenterology defines constipation as having less than three bowel movements per week as part of the diagnosis of IBS-C.[32] Based on our body's need to detoxify daily, I consider anything less than one bowel movement daily is as constipation.

Indigenous cultures who have lived off fresh, local, unprocessed diets can regularly have a bowel movement after each meal.[33] [34] Babies who are breastfed can have bowel movements once to several times a day. Note though that breast-fed babies may also not move their bowels daily. This is not considered constipation unless the stools are dry and hard or are difficult to pass.

There is a system in place in your body called the gastro-colic reflex (gastro= stomach and colic = colon) that links the eating and defecation process. When food enters your stomach and stretches it, a signal is sent to the small intestine and colon to increase movement there. The movement increases substantially in the sigmoid colon which is the part right before the rectum. When the pressure increases here, the reflex acts as a stimulus for defecation. This occurs due to the release of neuropeptides including serotonin, cholecystokinin, and gastrin. It has the effect of moving the bowels within as little as 15 minutes of eating.

Then why don't we all move our bowels after a meal? Because the system may not be working perfectly. Digestion is complex and multifactorial, and any number of factors can interfere with regular function. The same elements that cause IBS/SIBO can be the cause of constipation.

Some infants have a tendency towards constipation from birth. Often this is because of a food they are getting either directly or from nursing that their body does not work well with. There have been hundreds of times that a patient has told me they've been constipated since childhood and then their other digestive symptoms began to stack onto that as the years have gone by.

I love to treat babies and infants using my selective food introduction when their parents bring them in for symptoms of chronic constipation, colic, ear aches, rashes/eczema, re-occurring colds or congestion. Recurring, severe infections that have resulted in repeat antibiotic use and trips to urgent care can stop or decrease substantially when the underlying problem is a food that is irritating the developing digestive and immune system. It's a miracle to witness first-hand the power of removing the offending foods and watching their little immune systems bounce back in strength.

If there is a food we are eating – let's say it's cow dairy, and our body doesn't like it – it will let us know. It will tell us with nausea, vomiting, gas, stomach aches, diarrhea or even constipation. If we continue to eat this food and ignore these messages, then the body may or may not stop telling us that there is a problem with these symptoms; however, the problem remains. It may manifest later in life an unrelated immune compromise such as chronic sinusitis, a skin disorder or any number of deeper, delayed problems that interfere with the immune system. [35]

13.1.1 Treatment of Acute Constipation

Once more serious reasons for constipation have been ruled out, treatment of acute constipation includes increasing fiber, water or fluid intake and exercise. Patients are encouraged to avoid postponing bowel movements when the urge is present. This is especially true for children. Children are often misdiagnosed with encopresis or constipation when they are holding in their stools either because they are painful to pass or because they do not want to stop their current activity to use the toilet.

If this does not resolve acute symptoms, the next step would be adding bulk laxatives (psyllium, methylcellulose, prunes or over the counter stool softeners). If these are ineffective, the next step would be osmotic laxatives (magnesium or polyethylene glycol/MiraLAX) and finally stimulant laxatives (Bisacodyl). Other higher options include the use of linaclotide and lubiprostone. There is also a medication for constipation that occurs due to use of opioid pain treatments called Relistor, which is effective for people on these medications.

Travel-based constipation is a phenomenon that has interested me over the years. Many people experience a change in bowel movements when they travel or even spend the night in a new place. It doesn't seem to matter if time zone or diet remains the same – some people know they will struggle with constipation regardless. This suggests that the nervous system must be involved, and the stress of change (even good stress) can affect digestion.

For travel constipation, I recommend taking a laxative prior to going to bed on your first night, or first few nights that you are away. It just makes the whole experience more pleasant when regularity is not a concern. Your treatment may be as simple as magnesium or over the counter laxatives. If you have the time and resources, take some prunes, figs or chia pudding the first night and drink a cup of hot water with the juice of a fresh lemon in the morning.

13.1.2 Natural treatments for acute constipation

If you want to address acute constipation naturally, there are many choices. First, tend to your diet. Animal products like meats, cheese and dairy can slow the peristaltic movement. White flour, sugar and processed foods have very little fiber (or nutrients) so they do not help the bowels to move. The foods that will help your bowels to move are fruits, vegetables and whole grains. These are also called plant-based foods. It is important to listen to your urges and do not ignore the normal impulse to have a bowel movement. Do not rush your bowel movements. Doing so can lead to chronic constipation issues for children or adults. Chronic constipation can occur because the stagnation of constipation fills and distends the colon, which results in a loss of muscle tone and the impulse to empty the bowel can weaken.

Bulking fibers like chia or psyllium can be soaked in hot water and taken at bedtime. Mild herbal treatments like dandelion root, yellow dock or fennel seed can be made into teas which will stimulate bile and help the bowels to move. Herbs that relax the spasms in the colon include catnip, hops, lemon balm or chamomile. These can also be used in tea, tincture or glycerite form. Hot water and lemon contain limonene, which is a motility agent to move the system. This is a good morning drink. Another favorite, especially for children, is to massage warm castor oil into the abdomen at bedtime. Adding a couple drops of essential oil of lobelia, rosemary or lavender can be relaxing and helpful.

A squatting position when defecating can be very helpful to straighten the sigmoid colon, which is right before the rectum. Many cultures normally squat for bowel movements.

Straightening the sigmoid (an "S" shaped tube) into a more linear shape can reduce the pressure in the system and lessen the occurrence of diverticular disease from straining constipation. This position makes the stools easier to pass and can be especially helpful if the elasticity of the colon has been compromised.

I had the pleasure of treating a delightful 81-year-old man who reported that his symptoms started in 1969 following a surgery that removed his pyloric sphincter. The pyloric sphincter is the one-way valve that separates the stomach and the small intestine. With the pyloric valve gone, he had to sleep sitting up or bile would reflux up into his throat and cause burning. Sleeping in an upright position also lessened the fluid from accumulating in his stomach which gave him a sea-sick feeling. When he lay down, he said that it felt like his stomach was filling up at night and the fluid was sloshing around. Because of this, he was not able to eat much, and he had lost a lot of weight.

He had had many studies done with his gastroenterologist, including pH testing, gastric emptying, colonoscopies, and CT scans. His gastroenterologist had attempted a pyloric repair surgery, which was unsuccessful.

He also told me that he was very gassy and had extreme constipation that was not responding well to his use of stool softeners or propylene glycol. We talked about the anatomy of the digestive system and how it is really one continuous hose that runs for about thirty feet through the body. If the exit is not working well, then there will be back-pressure in the system, and that may be the cause of the fluid moving upwards and filling his stomach, regardless of the status of the pyloric sphincter. I started him on magnesium oxide, along with his existing constipation medications, GI Jan-aloe for the reflux, and GI Janel Digest B formula to improve the gastro-colic signals and assist his bowels to move. He had previously been avoiding both cow diary and gluten. We tested for food intolerances and gluten was not a problem, so I had him put that back in his diet. We found an overgrowth of candida in the stool and I treated him with a course of Diflucan.

By this time his bowels were beginning to move on a regular basis. We did a SIBO breath test and his results showed a single peak of hydrogen gas after 20 minutes, which reflects potential bacterial overgrowth in the stomach and the first part of the small intestine. I asked him to begin to take GI Janel One for digestive repair and SIBO. Once he added this into his protocol, the need to sleep sitting up began to lessen. He reported that his stomach filling and sloshing was subsiding, and the bile reflux into his throat had stopped. I had him do some visceral massage with our therapist who taught him how to massage his abdomen at home for regularity. He then found a therapist who taught him additional points on his body to massage which helped move his bowels. By this time, he was consistently sleeping in bed and enjoying his gluten breads. He continued a maintenance dose of GI Janel One, his digestive B formula, and GI Jan-aloe. With his bowels moving well, his upper digestive symptoms remain resolved.

13.2 DIARRHEA

Diarrhea is one of the methods your body has of rapidly eliminating an irritation. When a food irritates the intestine, diarrhea may occur immediately or, in the case of delayed reactions, even days later. Add to this the fact that your body may be irritated by more than one food type. If this is the case, then your diarrhea may be continuous due to continuous exposure to these irritating foods.

Diarrhea can also occur due to infections in the digestive system. Infections are caused by a bacteria, parasite or virus. Symptoms can be acute and pass within 24-48 hours. For example, acute food poisoning can occur when you eat food that has been sitting out for too long, like potato salad at a picnic. Symptoms may also be chronic and undiscovered by standard stool testing. Standard stool testing is becoming more comprehensive; however, it can still miss chronic, nonpathogenic bacteria or potentially pathogenic species that are causing the symptoms. Conventional lab tests for diarrhea do not examine the full spectrum of species in the microbiome.

A quick and easy resolution of chronic diarrhea can happen when we test the microbiome, find the problem, and give a course of appropriate antibiotics. I've seen this work well over and over. For children, a course of probiotics to stop the chronic diarrhea due to microbiome imbalance is also very effective.

Sometimes a person can be perfectly fine and healthy, but after dealing with an acute viral or bacterial diarrhea, things never quite go back to how there were. This is because the infection has caused a shift in the system that needs to be strengthened and repaired. It can be that the extra bit of stress caused by the infection starts a plethora of food sensitivities that were previously below the threshold of symptom expression. It is also suspected that an acute infection can damage the MMC (migrating motor complex). The term for this phenomenon is post infectious IBS or post infectious SIBO.

Diarrhea can also be the result of a trigger that may or may not even be present any longer. We call this molecular mimicry. For example, an acute episode of travelers' diarrhea will move through the body in hours or days. The infection is gone, but the diarrhea cycle may persist because the body has gone into a chronic inflammatory response. In a case like this, the immune system cannot turn off and continues to react as if the infection was still present.

For some people, diarrhea may even be a result of loss of tolerance to the normal microbiome. It is possible that this triggering has a strong role in chronic colitis (microscopic, lymphocytic, collagenous) or Inflammatory Bowel Disease (Crohn's and Ulcerative Colitis).

Diarrhea is categorized as either loose stools, frequent stools or both. Diarrhea can be a result of increased secretion of fluid into the intestine, decreased absorption from the intestine, or a rapid passage through the intestine. Often there is cramping pain that precedes the diarrhea, and there may be some relief following a bowel movement. There may be symptoms of stool incontinence, extreme urgency or incomplete evacuation where there is a need to return repeatedly to the toilet.

Absolute diarrhea is defined as more than five bowel movements a day. *Relative diarrhea* is an increase in frequency relative to an individual's typical number of daily bowel movements and increased loosening of the stool.

The dangers of chronic diarrhea are dehydration and an imbalance in electrolytes. Either of these can be very serious and require urgent care. Irritation to the anus can also occur with ongoing diarrhea.

Standard laboratory's tests for diarrhea include stool culture and microscopic testing for bacteria, parasites and white blood cells. Newer lab tests are employing PCR DNA or RNA analysis that will allow the lab to pick up virus, bacteria and parasites in one sample. Polymerase Chain Reaction (PCR) is a technique that allows a very tiny sample to be amplified for detection. Because these tests are new, the cost can be high if your insurance company does not cover them.

Functional labs will test for probiotic bacteria, potential pathogens, viruses, nonpathogens, yeasts and parasites as well as some measurements of digestion (food breakdown) and absorption (food transport from the intestinal tube into the body). This remains my preferred testing in terms of its ability to identify the problems that can be treated to resolve symptoms of chronic diarrhea for colitis and IBS-D/SIBO patients.

> *Here is a case where functional stool testing saved the day. A few years ago, I saw a 27-year-old mother who had a recent history of taking many courses of metronidazole for suspected bacterial vaginosis infections. Since these exposures, she had developed chronic diarrhea and upper right quadrant pain. An ultrasound of her gallbladder revealed sludge but not stones in the gallbladder. The stool testing that was done with her PCP showed no parasites or diarrhea causing bacteria in the standard lab panel. She had already removed many foods from her diet, including all the classic trigger foods for IBS/SIBO, but symptoms persisted. Based on her symptoms, I suspected that the internal lining of her*

digestive tract was too inflamed to handle any of the GI Janel Digest formulas, so I put her on the repair phase with GI Janel Aloe and GI Janel One only.

Her abdominal pain improved on this treatment, but the diarrhea was persistent and worsening to the point where she was waking at night several times with diarrhea. I requested that she use a low-fat diet based on her gallbladder findings, but this did not change the symptoms. We ran a SIBO breath test, which was negative, and then ran a functional stool test. The stool test was positive for an overgrowth of Citrobacter amalonaticus and Candida dubliniensis. The Citrobacter was sensitive to several of the antibiotics that the lab tested it for. We chose to use tetracycline for fourteen days combined with 200 billion flora daily. Since using an antibiotic will increase yeast overgrowth, I requested to see her after the course of this treatment to determine if we also needed to address the Candida (yeast) from the test results.

She came in after the fourteen days and had the most amazing report for me. The tetracycline had cleared all diarrhea after the third day of taking it. She was having 1-3 formed bowel movements a day, no gas, no reflux, no abdominal pain and no diarrhea. She then began adding foods back into her diet and found that there was nothing that she did not tolerate. If we did not do the functional stool testing, we never would have found the Citrobacter as this is not a bacterium that is reported on a standard stool panel. We also would not have known the correct antibiotic to use in order to remove the Citrobacter from her digestive system.

Imaging tests may be ordered for chronic diarrhea and these include barium x-rays, EGD (endoscope) colonoscopy, MRI enterography and CT imaging. Also helpful are SIBO tests, lactose or fructose intolerance tests, fat absorption tests and pancreatic testing.

Diarrhea can originate in the colon (large intestine) as IBD (ulcerative colitis), microscopic colitis (lymphocytic and collagenous), viral, bacterial or parasitic infections, eosinophilic colitis, ischemic colitis and malignancy.

Diarrhea can originate in the small intestine as Celiac disease (gluten), IBD (Crohn's disease), bile salt malabsorption, Brush border enzyme deficiency of lactase, sucrase or maltase, SIBO, radiation damage, overuse of NSAIDs (Ibuprofen, aspirin, naproxen, Celebrex), some cancers, tropical sprue and impaired lymphatic drainage. The most common form of chronic diarrhea in IBS-D/SIBO or IBS -M involves a food intolerance as part of the problem (or as the entire problem).

Diarrhea is classified as functional (multi-system and multi-factorial) in IBS and SIBO.

Diarrhea can have a systemic etiology from drugs, alcohol, advanced liver disease, immune deficiencies or amyloidosis.

Gastric bypass surgery, fecal impaction and pancreatic deficiency may result in chronic diarrhea.

The endocrine system causes of diarrhea include hyperthyroid disease, diabetes, hypo-parathyroid, Addison disease, gastrinoma, carcinoid tumors and VIPomas.

Foods that cause diarrhea can be any foods that you have become sensitized or intolerant to. Common food triggers include gluten, dairy, eggs, fried foods, citrus, excess fruits, rich and fatty foods, and alcohol-based sugars.

13.2.1 Acute treatment of diarrhea

For acute diarrhea symptoms, rehydration and use of electrolytes are important to keep the body hydrated. Over-the-counter bismuth products and products that slow motility can also be helpful. Until recently, conventional diets for diarrhea included the B.R.A.T diet (banana, rice, applesauce, toast), but that is currently considered overly restrictive.

13.2.2 Natural Treatments for Acute Diarrhea

Natural treatments include high-dose probiotics (200 billion or more organisms daily). I have listed my preferred probiotics for diarrhea symptoms in the appendix of this book.

Digestive teas, cold teas or punches of catmint, lemon balm, linden flowers, oats, skullcap and chamomile can be helpful for acute symptoms. Digestive enzymes and antimicrobial formulas with Cranesbill, Hydrastis, Althea and Bromelain are my favorites for travelers' diarrhea or acute food poisoning. Carob, acacia, activated charcoal, cinnamon and bentonite clay can also be used to slow down the bowels.

Styptic herbs like geranium and Achillea can be helpful, and I have used these in some cases of IBS/SIBO/IBD.

Diets should temporarily eliminate dairy and gluten, and promote easily-digested broths, rice and well-cooked vegetables or blended vegetable soups, bland chicken and fish, bananas and bland gluten free crackers and breads.

13.3 ABDOMINAL PAIN

From the extensive information listed below, you will see that there are many causes of abdominal pain. It is important that the serious causes are ruled out when diagnosing and treating this symptom. Valuable life-saving time can be wasted if you attempt to treat a serious cause of abdominal pain as if it were a functional diagnosis like IBS/SIBO. I encourage a full medical workup to exclude urgent and secondary causes of gastrointestinal pain prior to treatment with GI Janel formulas.

13.3.1 Abdominal Pain associated with IBS/SIBO

Pain can occur anywhere along the digestive tract. The most common pains that I see in general practice related to IBS/SIBO are listed below. I have summarized common digestive pains and pain that must be ruled out or treated as urgent concerns.

Esophagus – The most common pains are the result of burning or spams in the esophagus caused by gastric reflux (heartburn) and esophageal spasms or strictures. Lower esophageal sphincter pain arises from gastric reflux, hiatal hernia and LES (lower esophageal) valve defects.

Stomach – Burning pain can come from hyperacidity, H pylori infections, gastritis or ulcers. For a stomach ulcer (gastric ulcer), the burning is worse with food because this is when stomach acid is released. Bloating pains are common in IBS/SIBO due to food intolerances or bacterial and yeast overgrowth. In the cases of bacterial or yeast overgrowth in the stomach, there can be immediate bloating and distention on eating or drinking.

Small Intestine – Cramping or bloating pains can occur anywhere in the 25-foot-long small intestine. Generally, cramping pains are stimulated by food intolerances and bloating pains by overgrowth or infections. Sometimes, both cramping and bloating pain occur simultaneously. Bloating pain can be extreme and cause great pain, or it can distend the abdomen and be uncomfortable but not painful.

Colon – Cramping or bloating pains can be experienced in the large intestine (colon) for the same reasons as in the small intestine. Pain from infection of the appendix typically begins in the middle of the abdomen and radiates to the lower right corner. Lower left pain is most frequently caused by diverticulitis, especially in patients over 40 years of age. Upper right pain occurs frequently where the colon takes a 90-degree turn under the liver (hepatic flexure), while upper left pain occurs where the colon takes a second 90-degree turn under the spleen (splenic flexure). Upper right-sided abdominal pain is also commonly caused by gallbladder problems including inflammation, sludge or bile stones.

Rectum – Hemorrhoids and fissures result in itchy or burning pains that can worsen with diarrhea, constipation and straining. These may cause bright red blood in the stool or when you wipe.

13.3.2 Emergency Abdominal Pain

The follow is a list of acute causes of abdominal pain that require urgent care:

Obstructions – Adhesions, strangulations, volvulus, intussusception, malignancy (cancer which can be in the esophagus, stomach, colon, rectum, pancreas, liver or biliary system).

Inflammation – Meckel diverticulitis, cholecystitis (gallbladder), acute pancreatitis, acute diverticulitis, appendicitis and uncontrolled ulcerative colitis or Crohn's disease.

Perforation – Gastric ulcer (stomach), duodenal ulcer (small intestine), perforation of the esophagus.

Since the reproductive system is in the pelvic basin with the digestive system, pain can occur in the lower abdomen/pelvis in the form of a ruptured ovarian cyst, ectopic pregnancy, ovarian torsion, endometriosis or pelvic inflammatory disease (sexually transmitted infections).

Vascular pain includes aortic dissection or rupture of the aorta, Ischemic colitis, acute mesenteric ischemia or infarction (loss of blood flow), mesenteric artery syndrome, splenic infarct or rupture, ischemic colitis, radiation enteritis and Budd-Chiari syndrome.

Metabolic abdominal pain from diabetic ketoacidosis is another urgent concern.

Pain originating from the kidney can occur in nephrolithiasis (stones) and chronic pyelonephritis.

13.3.3   Other causes of Abdominal Pain

Less urgent vascular causes of pain include hematomas (bruises) of the abdominal wall and sickle cell crisis.

Other causes of chronic abdominal pain that may require less urgent care are: subacute infection, psoas damage (muscle), neutropenic enterocolitis, chronic hepatitis, mild gastroenteritis, mild infectious colitis, uremia, hereditary Mediterranean fever, acute intermittent porphyria, Addison's disease, hypercalcemia, toxic exposures, heavy metal poisoning, narcotic withdrawal, testicular torsion, celiac disease (gluten), lactase deficiency, chronic pancreatitis, chronic cholecystitis or cholelithiasis (inflammation, sludge or stones), gastroparesis (slow stomach emptying), centrally mediated pain syndrome, narcotic bowel syndrome, abdominal migraine or paroxysmal nocturnal hemoglobinuria

13.3.4   Natural Treatment of Acute Abdominal Pain

My first line physical medicine treatment is the Castor Oil Pack. This may be your grandma's medicine, but it works and is very comforting for abdominal pain and for constipation. Therapeutic oils have been used for centuries to relieve pain and regenerate the body. These oils can penetrate the skin layers, entering the lymphatic channels (waste cleaning system) that surround the abdominal organs. Here the oils promote an increase in the activity and quantity of white blood cells (the immune protective cells or gastrointestinal lymphatic tissue (GALT). The lymphatic channels are then able to shunt chemical stagnation out of the area.

The oils additionally act as an anti-inflammatory and can reduce chemical pain messengers, soothe damage and promote deep healing. When applied to the liver, there is an increase in activity of detoxification and liver regeneration. This is a lipoatrophic effect, assisting the liver to remove toxins from your body. [36]

For babies and infants (who are not constipated), I prefer to treat acute abdominal pain with simple catnip tea or peppermint tea, or punch sweetened with honey or loquat syrup.

Even for adults, sipping strong peppermint, spearmint or catmint tea can be helpful for gastrointestinal (GI) pain. Other herbs for relief of GI pain are hops, lemon balm, anise, cardamom, cinnamon, cloves or meadowsweet. Capsule versions of herbs in the essential oil form can be helpful for acute abdominal pain but are often too strong and irritating for IBS/SIBO patients.

Peppermint oil is offered as a natural product for intestinal spasm, but I have seen very limited success with this in my practice. The side effects include peppermint burping which can also irritate patients who have concomitant reflux disease. The oils can irritate the lower part of the intestines as they move through the body. The problem here is that most patients with IBS/SIBO already have weakened and irritated digestive systems. Peppermint oils are often too strong to use without side effects.

Peppermint is relatively safe to ingest. There are, however, volatile (essential or aromatic) oils which contain chemicals that can be toxic to the body and should not be ingested.

13.4 BLOATING

There are several reasons for bloating in an IBS/SIBO patient. The reasons may appear to be individual problems, but more commonly they exist simultaneously. They include food irritations, hypochlorhydria (low stomach acid output), hypofunction of the exocrine pancreas (Exocrine Pancreas Insufficiency or EPI) gallbladder insuficiency, functional damage of the intestinal (GI) barrier, chronic infections like SIBO (bacterial overgrowth in the small intestine), SIFO (small intestinal fungal overgrowth), or chronic dysbiosis of the microbiome in the large intestine (colon). Underlying damage to the intestinal cells must be resolved to permanently strengthen the system and prevent the return of IBS/SIBO symptoms.

Bloating and gas always come from bacteria, yeast or other species that live inside your digestive system. Your body does not make the gas. The organisms consume your food and release gas as a part of their process. This may or may not be an overgrowth issue.

Ongoing irritation by food and hidden infections will affect the gastrointestinal barrier. This in turn, can lead to bloating symptoms, even if there is no overgrowth of bacteria or yeast in the small intestine.

Remember that the tube of the small intestine is made of cells with a basement membrane wrapping. The cells fold in on themselves to make an enormous surface area for the absorption of nutrients. These folds look like the bristles of a brush. We call this internal surface the brush border.

Small Intestine
Wall Details

Small Intestine Cross Section
Brush Border

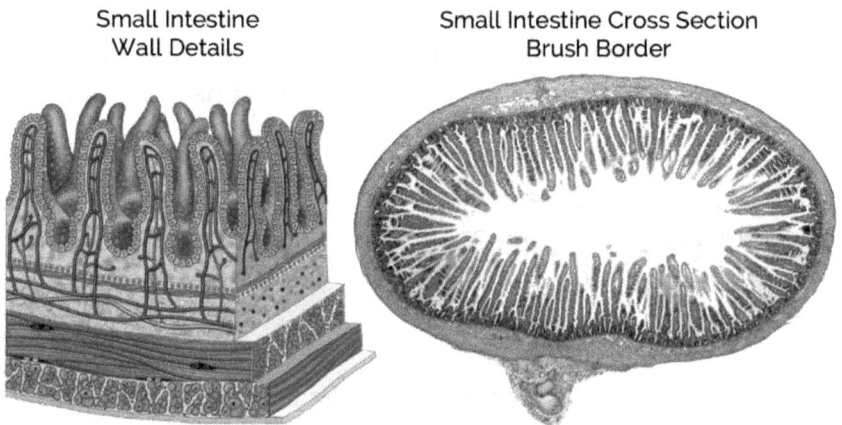

Figure 13.1 Brush Border – Cross Section

The projections on top of the intestinal cell that make the brush border are called *villi*. The villi and brush border are covered with a mucous layer that has many crucial protective functions. All together this system is the gastrointestinal barrier that separates the outside of the body (inside the digestive tube) from the inside of the body. This mucus layer protects the brush border, allows the food to move more easily through the tube, and is the home of beneficial bacteria (also call the microbiome).

When sugars (carbohydrates) and proteins arrive at the small intestine for absorption, they have been broken down by pancreatic enzymes, but are still not completely ready to cross the gastrointestinal barrier. They must be broken down from di-peptides (two peptides or protein building blocks) and disaccharides (two sugar building blocks) into single units. Only the monosaccharide and monopeptide (amino acid) can be transported across a healthy gastrointestinal barrier. The final digestive enzymes for carbohydrate breakdown are called disaccharidases (they break apart two connected sugar molecules).

This is another really important element to understanding the symptoms of IBS/SIBO. The healthy intestinal cell is where these disaccharidases and dipeptidases are manufactured and released.

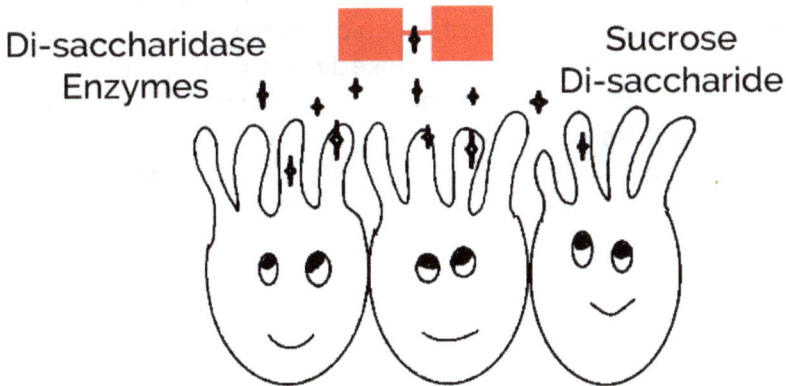

Figure 13.2 Disaccharide cleavage and absorption. Carbohydrates and proteins are digested along their travel in the intestine. In order to cross the Gastrointestinal Barrier, they must be split into single units (monosaccharides and amino acids). Healthy small intestinal cells manufacture and release the final

digestive enzymes for the breakdown of carbohydrates and proteins.

The job of the gastrointestinal barrier enzymes is to break apart carbohydrates, which are made of two building blocks (disaccharides). This results in two monosaccharides that can then be picked up by receptors on the intestinal cell surface. The cell can then transport the monosaccharide through itself and into the body. If these enzymes are missing due to microscopic damage, then the carbohydrates cannot be transported by the cell. They will subsequently sit in the intestine and become food for the bacteria and yeast that live there. That bacteria and yeast consume the carbohydrate and produce gas.

Do you see how most of the low-carb IBS/SIBO diets work? Diets like the SCD, FODMAP, SIBO and Gaps eliminate the fermentable carbohydrates from the diet. If there is nothing to ferment, you will have less gas.

This condition is also known as carbohydrate intolerance. If disaccharides cannot be broken down, they will be unable to pass through the gastrointestinal barrier into the blood stream for the body to use. Instead, they will sit in the small intestine and form gas by fermentation because they are acting as food for intestinal bacteria or yeast. If you combine yeast and sugar, you will make gas. If you've ever baked bread you know what happens when you add sugar to yeast. It rises in a gassy blob, doubling or tripling in size. People who have the bloating and gassiness associated with IBS/SIBO are very familiar with this and can probably picture it happening inside.

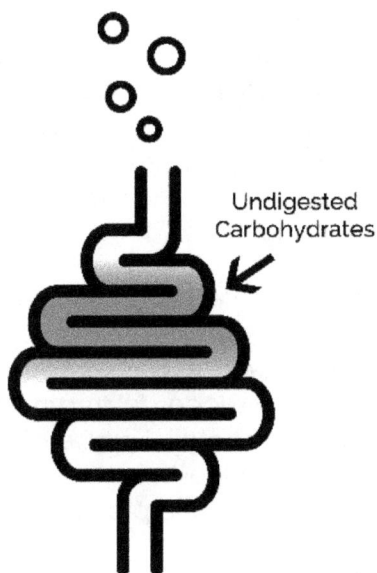

Figure 13.3 *Intestinal Gas created by undigested carbohydrates.*

When a patient tells me that they have reduced digestive symptoms on one of the low carbohydrate diets (SCD, FODMAP, GAPS, Paleo, Ketogenic, SIBO), this is an important clue for me! This means that there is a problem due to the fermentation of sugars (disaccharides), but not necessarily bacterial or yeast overgrowth. We then start to repair the problem so that carbohydrates can ultimately be added back in the diet.

I don't find low carbohydrate diets necessary. Where I've seen most improvement for hundreds of patients, is to run an IgG food panel or do a diet elimination and determine the specific foods which are inflammatory to the patient. These foods must be avoided to stop the chronic inflammation that they are triggering. I have my patients avoid their IgG restrictions and add the carbohydrates back, along with supplements to support the digestive health. Many times, this resolves bloating symptoms on its own by allowing the body to come back into its natural homeostasis.

My point is that if you only restrict fermentable foods, and do not address the other inflammatory foods of repair of the system, then the weakness perpetuates and the chances of bacterial or yeast overgrowth and bloating returning are very likely.

This is a different approach than the current SIBO treatment, which focuses on infection and motility issues. What I have found is that when we remove irritating foods that may or may not be carbohydrate-based and support digestion, for most patients the symptoms resolve, and then the body can take care of any SIBO itself. Additionally, motility issues are resolved when digestion is no longer being constantly irritated by inflammatory food.

Remember, IBS/SIBO bloating is not an isolated disorder with a single cause. It is a part of the IBS complex of defects. Here's how I look at it: Is SIBO the cause, or the result, of the problem? In my opinion and in my experience after many successful treatments, I am convinced that SIBO is the result. This bacterial proliferation in the small intestine can add to the existing digestive symptoms; however, it is rarely (possibly never) a standalone problem.

Bloating can be experienced as a distention of the abdomen that occurs in episodes, or it can exist as a symptom that is always present. It may worsen during the day, resolve overnight, and then return the following day. Bloating can also be very painful for some patients who are unable to release the gas, and who have cramping occurring with the bloating digestive tract.

Ovarian cancer also has symptoms of lower abdominal pain and bloating and can mimic those of IBS/SIBO. This is an important rule-out diagnosis that can be missed and assumed to be IBS/SIBO. Your doctor may send you for imaging test or do a blood test called CA-125 to rule this out.

13.4.1 Natural Treatment for Bloating and Gas

If bloating, distention, or gassy pain is your primary symptom, and if life-threatening causes for it have been ruled out, see my section on fast tracking GI Janel One for permanent relief. That is my best recommendation.

Charcoal can be used acutely as a binder for occasional bloating symptoms or in the initial stages of treatment. It will not solve the problem of IBS/SIBO, but it can give symptomatic relief.

For some people with less complicated symptoms of IBS/SIBO, using the GI Janel Digest (A, B or C) formulas will be enough to manage bloating symptoms. If this is the case for you, what it means is that your primary issue is digestive reserve and you lack the ability to release adequate gastric acid, pancreatic enzymes or bile to fully digest your food.

14 SIBO

It is estimated that 50-70% of IBS patients have SIBO. However, SIBO is not a standalone diagnosis. Therefore, SIBO patients are cautioned that the symptoms can return anytime. SIBO and IBS are overlapping and must be treated together for permanent symptom resolution.

I am listing SIBO under the symptom heading in this book because it does not occur alone but is a part of the IBS spectrum. SIBO is not the cause of your symptoms. SIBO is a result of gastrointestinal barrier breakdown (leaky gut), food intolerance and system deficiency. If these causes are not addressed, symptoms can and will easily return even after antibiotic or antimicrobial treatment. The GI Janel system works to repair the gastrointestinal barrier, resolve local motility and support system deficiency. All you must do is remove the offending foods, then gradually add them back as tolerated once you are stronger.

SIBO or small intestinal bacterial overgrowth has received a lot of press lately. With the promotion of Xifaxan (rifaximin), you can now find copious advertising information about treating IBS-D related symptoms with this antibiotic. Xifaxan is approved by the FDA for use in IBS-D. This treatment is helpful for some, and for others gives a temporary relief. When symptoms are relieved on a medication but then return when off the medication, it means the cause of the problem is still there. In integrative medicine, we are trained to "treat the cause" of disease. In fact, this is one of the principles of the study of naturopathic medicine:

Identify and Treat the Causes (Tolle Causam)

The naturopathic physician seeks to identify and remove the underlying causes of illness if possible, and reserves suppression of symptoms for when necessary.

Classic SIBO occurs when there is a backflow from the large intestine to the small intestine or following an acute gastrointestinal infection. Since the large and the small intestine have completely different microbiomes, physiologies and functions, we do not want to have their bacteria mixing. SIBO can also occur when the normal bacterial (or yeast) population of the small intestine overgrows in a weakened digestive system. SIBO can also occur when bacteria or yeast eaten with food (remember food is NOT sterile) are able to grow in the small intestine. This will occur with digestive reserve deficiencies in the stomach, pancreas or gall bladder. This deficiency can also be a result of long-term suppression of stomach acidity by acid-blocking drugs. This is the rationale for using the GI Janel Digest Formulas, which support the work of the secondary digestive organs and the breakdown of food within the small intestine.

There is a one-way valve that connects the small intestine (where food is digested and absorbed) to the large intestine, which compacts the waste into feces. If the valve becomes faulty, microbes from the large intestine can flow backward into the small intestine. These microbes (bacteria) or yeasts are now in contact with food that they can metabolize (eat) to produce gas. The bacteria in the colon is normally much more plentiful than in the small intestine. In some cases, regardless of the type of bacteria, simply the quantity of bacteria can be overwhelming and ferment the food in the small intestine before it is digested and absorbed into the body. Killing these extra bacteria with antibiotics will not address the underlying problem of the valve defect, motility issues or gastrointestinal barrier repair.

Right colic

Transverse colon

Left colic

Descending colon

Ascending colon

Epiploic appendages

Ileum

Tenia coil

Ileocecal sphincter (valve)

Haustra

Cecum

Rectum

Vermiform appendix

Anal canal

Mesoappendix

Anus

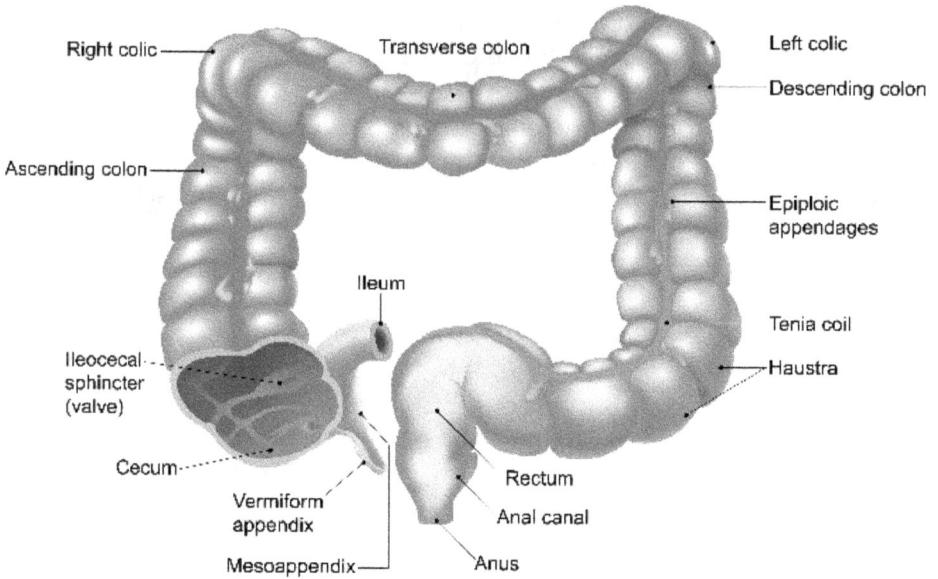

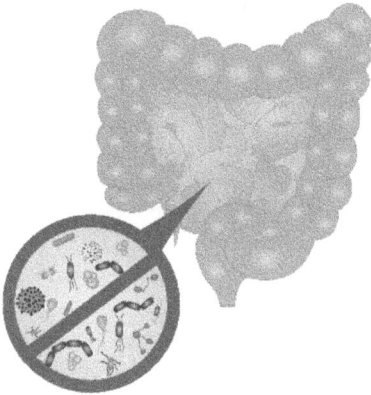

Figure 14.1 *A damaged ileocecal valve can permit backflow of bacteria from the large to the small intestine.*

SIBO is less likely to occur for people who have had their appendix removed. The appendix contains bacteria that may function to re-populate the intestine following infection. If the gastrointestinal barrier is strong, having an intact appendix should not be a problem. If the gastrointestinal barrier is weak or compromised, SIBO is more likely to occur and the bacteria from the appendix can accelerate the overgrowth.

These is also some new research by the neurologist Stasha Gominiack MD, indicating that Vitamin D levels greater than 55 ng/dl are required for the desired commensal bacteria to dominate in the small intestine rather than the SIBO organisms. [37]

Using antibiotics, it is possible to kill the SIBO bacteria, but not selectively. This means that the good bacteria die with the bad. Bacteria that is good in the large intestine but bad in the small intestine can be killed in both areas. There is a population of bacteria and yeasts that normally live in the small intestine. These can also be killed by the SIBO antibiotic. In the large intestine, there is also a normal population of yeast. There are up to 10,000 yeast organisms per gram of stool in a healthy body.

Antibiotic treatment for SIBO is a solution, I'll give you that. However, if we were to *repair* the system, support the digestive process, eliminate irritants and bring the body back into homeostasis (which is the state of natural health), then symptoms of SIBO could resolve without antibiotics and remain that way.

> *An entire family of four was referred to me by a colleague. They had been diagnosed with SIBO, and their diet was very restrictive when I first saw them. They all reported symptoms of alternating diarrhea and constipation along with abdominal pain, bloating and bad breath. No family members could tolerate diary, eggs, legumes, wheat or coffee without worsening symptoms. They were treated three years prior with a course of Xifaxan, which was followed by a gluten-free diet. The SIBO symptoms returned ten months later, at which time they were all given a second course of Xifaxan, followed by the SCD (specific carbohydrate diet). A few months later, they attempted to expand their SCD to include more carbohydrates. At this point they all regressed back to their IBS/SIBO symptoms and their tests were positive for SIBO again. This was when they came in to see me. When we first met, their diet was limited to beef, fish, lettuce, greens, carrots, rice, citrus, banana and berries.*

> *We immediately began food desensitization along with GI Janel Digest B and GI Janel One at gradually increasing doses. I saw them all eight weeks later and while their diet*

was the same, they all gave reports of improved GI symptoms including less gas, bloating, pain and constipation or diarrhea. I kept them on the GI Janel formulas until their next visit. Eight weeks later, they began to experiment with foods. They added back legumes, buckwheat and dairy and all tolerated this well. We also discussed adding in a tea of fennel, anise, caraway and clove for motility at the request of the patients. Following this their diets again were able to be expanded, to the point where they could eat all foods, including gluten. They were even tolerating sugar well. I continued to follow them at eight-week intervals, to permanently desensitize their food reactions, and we have not had a symptoms recurrence of SIBO or IBS since.

Xifaxan has been approved by the FDA for the treatment of IBS-D but not for SIBO. Xifaxan is being marketed for use with IBS-D. The FDA has not yet approved Xifaxan for use in SIBO. The standard treatment is a course of 550 mg taken three times a day for 14 days. The course of antibiotics can be repeated up to 2 more times following the initial dose. Studies done on the drug show that symptom relief can last up to 6 months following treatment with Xifaxan.

Remember when we were talking about the healing wisdom of your body? If you have IBS or SIBO and you hit that overgrowth hard with antibiotics, you may be causing more harm than good. Currently, the antibiotic Xifaxan is off label use for SIBO. It is approved for use by the FDA as a treatment for IBS-D.

It seems to me that taking antibiotics for a system that depends on bacteria as its core function is not a promising idea. The manufacturer of Xifaxan contends that the antibiotic can discriminate between the beneficial bacteria that you want to keep in the large intestine and to a smaller degree in the small intestine. I have been assured by the pharmacy representatives that this is the case. I'm not convinced. If we kill the good with the bad there is a potential to further weaken an already compromised system. If you take a course of antibiotics and feel better and then the symptoms return, have you really treated the cause of the problem? *No, you have not.*

While I have no issues prescribing Xifaxan (especially if the patient really wants to try it), it is not the ultimate step in strengthening and repairing the system. That work still must be done to prevent symptom recurrence.

The cause of SIBO is a weakened digestive system that cannot keep the bacteria from the colon from back flowing or simply overgrowing in the small intestine. The system is hospitable to overgrowth of bacteria because of damage to the gastrointestinal barrier and valves.

GI Janel strengthens the cells of the digestive system and the gastrointestinal barrier so that the problem is resolved. Permanently.

As far as fungal overgrowth (SIFO), you should know that yeast is present in us and on us even when we are healthy. Most people think of this as Candida, but there are many different yeast species besides Candida. Some of this yeast is part of our normal protective flora. The human body carries ten times more microbial cells than human cells.[38] For the most part, we have a symbiotic relationship with these species when we have a strong immune defense system. In the case of fungal overgrowth (SIFO), as in the case of SIBO, if we strengthen the system and use GI Janel One as an antifungal and natural antibiotic therapy, the body takes care of the overgrowth and repair, and symptoms resolve. Yeast can also overgrow in the large intestine either with or without overgrowth in the small intestine. This exacerbates gassy symptoms of SIBO.

Remember that the body is striving to keep you heathy and vital. The vital force is strong if it has the nutrients it requires and is free of overwhelming irritation. Removing offending foods removes digestive irritation. The GI Janel formula repairs the cells, basement membrane and mucous lining of the digestive tract. GI Janel One is a natural antibacterial and anti-fungal agent, so that even without antibiotics or antifungal medication, your symptoms will improve, and for many, will resolve.

Imagine living without episodes of painful gas and bloating regardless of what you want to eat? This is very possible.

> Here is an example of a 35-year-old patient that saw me for only three visits to alleviate her symptoms. She told me that she had over six years of gas distention and abdominal pain that worsened as the day went on. She could pass some gas but not enough for pain relief. She was constipated and moved her bowels only once every seven days, unless she took a laxative. With the laxative, she would eliminate with cramping movements several times until the effect of the laxative wore off. Her social activities were limited due to the constant pain. She found it difficult to be at work and she was at the end of her rope with these symptoms. She told me that she was isolating herself socially due to the embarrassment and pain.
>
> She had been to the gastroenterologist and like most SIBO patients, her colonoscopy was normal. She was already eating a diet that eliminated gluten, diary, whole egg, soy, nuts and shellfish, so there was no need for food testing. I gave her a SIBO test kit and asked her to start on GI Janel Digest A with meals, GI Janel One at ½ tsp per day and 900 mg of magnesium hydroxide twice daily, once she had collected her sample.
>
> She returned four weeks later and told me that all her bloating and gassiness were better and most days she was moving her bowels easily. Her SIBO was positive for both methane and hydrogen levels. I asked her to begin increasing her dose of GI Janel One gradually by ½ tsp each five days until she reached six heaping teaspoons, and to hold the dose there for eight weeks. She came in following this treatment and she reported a full resolution of her symptoms. She repeated her SIBO test which was then negative for overgrowth.

She scheduled a follow up in one year while staying on her digestive support and introducing foods back into her diet one at a time, each seven days. When I saw her one year later, she told me that she found her bowels slowed down with heavy gluten consumption, but she could have a little gluten with no symptoms. Other than that, she was able to integrate dairy, eggs and soy without problems. She continued to avoid the nuts and shellfish that she had IgE (immediate) hypersensitivity to.

14.1 MOTILITY

Killing any extra bacteria will not resolve the motility problems in the intestine. I do not believe that prescriptive motility agents are necessary or helpful. Lack of proper peristalsis or motility in the intestine can be a major factor in the stagnation that allows bacteria overgrowth. However, isolating motility in treatment is not enough. Every time I see a digestive patient, I listen to their abdominal sounds with my stethoscope. This is an important part of determining motility and the extent of the gas sounds, as well as predominant locations of gassiness or immobility.

The primary cause of the motility defect is inflammation in the GI tract. This leads us right back to removing the irritating foods that are causing inflammation, supporting digestion (GI Janel Digest: A, B or C), repairing the integrity of the gastrointestinal barrier, brush border and ileocecal valve (GI Janel One), and providing a rich ecosystem base for the balanced microbiome (GI Jan-Aloe)

I am willing to entertain that there may be additional damage to the migrating motor complex of the digestive system, but I believe these cases are few and far between. Why? Because without doing *anything* to directly influence the nervous system, I have seen my patients permanently resolve their SIBO issues by addressing the elements above.

With the GI Janel system, motility is regained by removing chronic inflammation caused by foods or infections and repairing the cell structure and function through nutrient based treatment in the form of GI Janel One.

Here's an example of motility recovery in a SIBO patient. A 50-year-old woman was referred to me by a local colleague. This lovely woman reported 20 years of gas pain episodes that lasted for 24 hours at a time. She said that these episodes were becoming more and more frequent. She saw a gastroenterologist in 2011, who tested her as negative for celiac disease (gluten) and found her otherwise normal. In 2016, her gastroenterologist had her try a FODMAP diet, which helped a little. Five months prior to her visit with me, she saw a different gastroenterologist who tested her for SIBO. Her SIBO test came back with high hydrogen gases from 90 to 135 minutes. This represents gas production from the end of the small intestine and into the colon. She was put on a course of Xifaxan, followed by a 3-month course of erythromycin for motility. Since her symptoms did not change with this treatment, she came to see me.

I requested that she follow my soft food diet and begin taking GI Janel Digest A at meals with a starting dose of ½ teaspoon of GI Janel One daily. We sent in a blood test for inflammatory foods. The blood test came back positive for whole eggs and cow diary. When she did an elimination and challenge with these two foods, she reported a noticeable increase in her symptoms when she ate eggs, mayonnaise and cow dairy. She then continued the soft food diet and removed dairy and eggs as these would cause bloating for up to 3 days after she consumed them. I asked her to gradually increase her dose of GI Janel One to 6 teaspoons daily, which is the therapeutic dose.

When we met four weeks later, she reported feeling better overall, but she continued to have afternoon episodes of bloating occasionally. I suspected that there was more than SIBO happening here, so we repeated her SIBO breath test. The test came back negative for bacterial gasses after being treated with 8-week course of GI Janel One. Since we know that a large majority of SIBO patients also have SIFO (fungal overgrowth), I asked her to take a *course of voriconazole, which is one of the newest antifungal agents. Her insurance company would not cover the cost of this, so I sent in a prescription for itraconazole. Her insurance company would not cover this either, so I asked her to take amphotericin B, which is only available through a compounding pharmacy. I requested that she take 250 mg of amphotericin B twice daily before lunch and dinner.*

Several weeks later, she messaged me that her symptoms were completely gone. Our plan was then to move to a maintenance dose of her supplements and eventually re-introduce egg and cow dairy to see if they continue to be problems. We did not use a motility agent. We did not have to. What we did do is remove her offending foods, supply her with nutrients to repair her system, and treat the underlying infection. Then, the motility took care of itself as it was no longer challenged by these other inflammatory issues. I highly suspect that will be the end of this problem for her.

14.2 SIBO GASSES

There are two types of gas produced in SIBO that can be tested: methane and hydrogen gas. Bacteria produce hydrogen (hydrogen dominant SIBO) and Archaea, a non-bacterial single cell organism, produce methane gas (methane dominant SIBO). Methanobrevibacter species can also produce methane gas. It is reported that hydrogen-dominant SIBO can typically produce diarrhea symptoms while methane-dominant SIBO can typically produce constipation. Both species may be present as the Archaea consume the hydrogen gas that the bacteria make and produce methane (which is flammable). Even though, it is reported that diarrhea and constipation are associated with the various gasses, I have rarely found this correlation in my clinical experience.

A third gas produced in SIBO is hydrogen sulfide. This gas is hot, smelly and creates a feeling of burning. I suspect that this gas is closer to the origin of SIBO symptoms than the other two. It is theorized by Dr. Greg Nigh, ND, that an increase in hydrogen sulfide producing bacteria is a compensation mechanism by the body to restore the body's depleted sulfur. He also suggests that the hydrogen sulfide gas is the upstream problem and that the methane and hydrogen production is dysbiosis as result of this underlying sulfur deficiency.[39] I believe he is correct.

One of the most important first steps in treating SIBO symptoms (gassiness) is improving the capacity to digest your food. Therefore, your very first treatment in the GI Janel line will be one of the digestive supports: GI Janel A, B or C as tolerated. (See chapters on dosing.)

For SIBO treatment, digestive support is imperative! If there is not adequate digestive reserve in the stomach, pancreas or gallbladder, food will not be broken down properly right from the beginning. This leaves food particles which can feed bacteria, increasing bacteria overgrowth. The bacteria ferment food particles, which then cause gas and pressure in the abdomen. The result is SIBO gas pain and gas distention. This gas can also impact reflux (heartburn), as it can push upwards. Have you ever burped (gas release) and experienced burning in your chest or throat? This type of heartburn is caused by gas, not fluid from the stomach. It may be a form of "silent reflux". One ounce of undigested carbohydrates can produce more than ten quarts of hydrogen gas in the intestine.[40] Ten quarts of gas in your abdomen can be very painful.

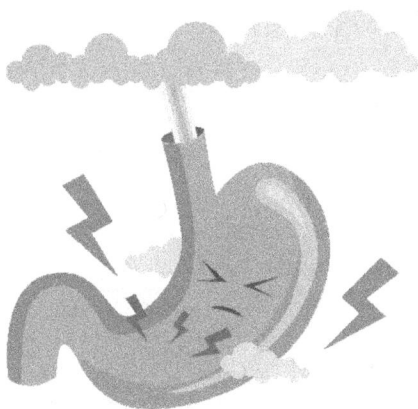

Figure 14-2 *Low acid and gas reflux. Proteins will not be broken down in low stomach acid. Undigested proteins will feed bacteria, resulting in bacterial overgrowth and gas production. They can move upward, causing upper gastrointestinal distention, gas pain, burping and gassy heartburn (reflux).*

14.3 NERVOUS SYSTEM AND SIBO

One way that GI Janel supports the nervous system is by restoring the body's deficiency of sulfur. It is plausible that Sulfur deficiency can impact GI motility, which is controlled by the nervous system. Our nervous system doesn't work properly if nerves cannot function properly or if neurotransmitters cannot be effectively broken down and removed or recycled. Our neurotransmitters will be inadequate to perform their motility functions with a deficiency of the nutrient Sulfur.

14.4 NATURAL MOTILITY TREATMENT SUMMARY

1. GI Janel Digestion Formula A, B or C to decrease the food source for SIBO, decrease SIBO species with food, and trigger the gastrocolic reflex

2. GI Janel One for repair of cellular structure, function and microbiome

3. GI Jan-Aloe for mucous layer repair

4. Remove offending foods

5. Remove unwanted yeasts, bacteria or parasites

6. GI Janel AM / BM, if required for regular, daily bowel movements

I rarely need to employ further treatments for motility. Your symptom relief will speak for itself. However here are some herbal options for initial treatment support, which can also be useful for digestive maintenance.

I prefer natural rather than prescription treatments for motility in the form of herbs. Teas or herbal punches (cold teas) work well for children or adults to soothe and gently assist motility.

Spearmint, peppermint, catnip, fennel, cardamom and anise are digestive herbs that are helpful for gassy symptoms and can support motility. The mint family (which includes catmint or catnip) is my favorite for the acute treatment of gassy nausea and abdominal pain. I will sometimes blend the herbs together or give warm catmint tea (Nepeta is the Latin name) by the spoonful to babies to settle their digestion. These are tasty teas that can be sipped throughout the day in the preliminary stages of your SIBO repair when you are still having symptoms. The peels of oranges or lemon contain a phytochemical terpene called D-Limonene which improves bowel motility. A tea with lemon and lemon peel or orange peel can be a gentle treatment for bowel motility. Ginger can also be used if tolerated, but not everyone has a strong enough digestive system for this herb.

There is some research from the neurologist Dr. Stasha Gominiack, MD that suggests that Vitamin D levels must be higher than 55 ng/dl for proper acetylcholine production.[41] This is significant because the Vagus nerve that instructs intestinal motility operates with the neurotransmitter acetylcholine. The enzyme which produces acetylcholine is vitamin D dependent. However, acetylcholine is an important neurotransmitter in many other parts of your body.

15 NON-INFLAMMATORY BOWEL DISEASE

Non-inflammatory bowel diseases are diagnosed based on the biopsy results following a colonoscopy (colon scope) or endoscopy.

The forms of non-inflammatory bowel disease include microscopic colitis (collagenous and lymphocytic colitis), ischemic colitis, segmental colitis associated with diverticula, radiation colitis, diversion colitis, eosinophilic colitis and Behcet's colitis.

The symptoms of non-inflammatory bowel disease overlap with IBS-D and with IBD (Inflammatory Bowel Disease: ulcerative colitis and Crohn's). Patients with non-inflammatory bowel disease report ongoing, uncontrollable diarrhea, cramping GI pain and bloating. Unlike inflammatory bowel disease patients, they do not exhibit blood in the stools other than a small amount of bright red bleeding from fissures at the anus.

Some medications have been associated with the onset of microscopic colitis. These include NSAIDs, heartburn medications and some antidepressants. Microscopic colitis is more common in woman and people older than 45 years. It also may have a genetic component and run in families.

There is a simple test to help differentiate inflammatory bowel disease from non-inflammatory disease and IBS. It is a stool sample called fecal calprotectin that can be performed at a standard lab.

Additional blood testing is available to rule out inflammatory bowel disease before sending a patient in for a colonoscopy or EGD. These blood tests look for antibodies to Saccharomyces cerevisiae (food or baker's yeast), atypical antineutrophil cytoplasmic antibodies, antichitobioside carbohydrate antibodies, antilaminaribioside carbohydrate antibodies, antimannobioside carbohydrate antibodies and atypical perinuclear antineutrophil cytoplasmic antibodies.

15.1 Treatments for Non-Inflammatory Bowel Disease

Standard conventional treatment includes the avoidance of dairy, caffeine and high fat foods, the addition of fiber supplementation and the use of over the counter medications like Imodium and Pepto-Bismol. Prescription drugs to reduce inflammation, such as mesalamine (Asacol, Canasa, Pentasa), sulfasalazine (Azulfidine), or steroids are sometimes prescribed.

Biologic drugs and other specific inflammatory inhibiting drugs are the most recent treatments for inflammatory bowel disease. These can be very helpful for the people who respond well to them. These are not yet approved treatments for non-inflammatory bowel disease.[42]

15.2 Natural Treatments for Non-Inflammatory Bowel Disease

Some of the principles for treating IBS-D/SIBO can be used to treat non-inflammatory bowel disease. The strongest correlation that I have seen clinically with the onset of non-inflammatory bowel disease has been the long-term use of oral antibiotics (over months or years). Typically, these have been prescribed for acne, rosacea or other skin problems. I have also seen non-inflammatory bowel disease manifest in patients with a history of infant exposure to repeated oral antibiotics (ear infections, tonsillitis, or strep throat).

Natural treatments for non-Inflammatory colitis can include fiber supplements and healing herbs like DGL (deglycyrrhizinated licorice) or Althaea (marshmallow root) and aloe inner fillet. There are also some specific probiotics that I will prescribe for acute and chronic diarrhea disorders.

Functional stool testing has helped many of my patients. It appears that the symptoms of microscopic colitis can be triggered by bacteria or yeast that may not be considered pathogenic species. These will not be reported on a conventional stool panel, but can be identified with functional stool testing, treated and eliminated to resolve the symptoms.

When these bacteria or yeast are identified in the stool, I prefer to prescribe antibiotics or prescription antifungals with high dose probiotics. This may seem counter-intuitive since antibiotics may have contributed to the problem in the first place, but since the symptoms can resolve quickly on this treatment after dealing with debilitating diarrhea for months or years, it just makes clinical sense. The functional labs will provide culture and sensitivity testing, so we can target exactly what to use to eradicate the microorganism. I have never had to repeat this antibiotic treatment if the digestive system is cleaned up and repaired following the antibiotic or antifungal use.

I have found allergy desensitization to be a successful treatment to calm down the chronic diarrhea and discomfort for non-IBD patients. You can read more about this therapy on my website, as it is not in the scope of this book.

I began prescribing my GI Janel One formula to both non-inflammatory and inflammatory bowel disease patients (Crohn's and ulcerative colitis). I was surprised to find these patients coming back reporting a normalization of stools and decreased pain. This indicates a sulfur deficiency and or a microbiome imbalance as an aspect of these disorders.

16 OTHER DIAGNOSES

16.1 CARBOHYDRATE INTOLERANCE

Just to drive this point home again, carbohydrate intolerance occurs at the level of the small intestinal cell just before the food is transported across the gastrointestinal barrier. Carbohydrates are made from sugar building blocks. The most concentrated carbohydrates are grains and sugars.

The pancreas releases enzymes that start to breakdown carbohydrates after the teeth have mashed them up. These enzymes are released in the small intestine. The pancreatic enzymes will not digest the carbohydrates all the way to monosaccharides (single sugars). The disaccharides (two connected sugar molecules) arriving at the small intestine cells cannot be taken from the intestine and into the body until they are chopped into two separate monosaccharide building blocks.

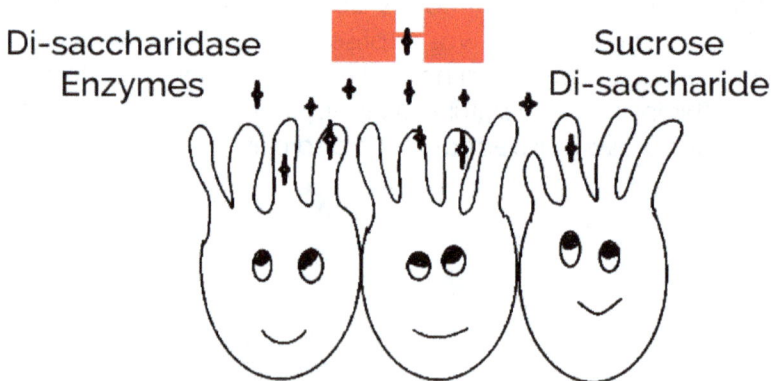

Figure 16.1 *Disaccharide enzymes break disaccharides into mono saccharides for transport into the body.*

Maltase disaccharidase splits maltose into two molecules of glucose.

Lactase disaccharidase splits lactose into a glucose molecule and a galactose molecule.

Sucrase disaccharidase splits sucrose into a glucose molecule and a fructose molecule.

If the disaccharides cannot be enzymatically cleaved into monosaccharides for transport into the body, they will sit in the intestine, unable to cross the gastrointestinal barrier. They are then susceptible to fermentation in the intestine, regardless of the number of bacteria present. The fermentation can occur with the normal bacteria or yeast that live in the small intestine or it can be increased when there is an increased population of bacterial or yeast in the small intestine (SIBO/SIFO).

The test for SIBO employs a synthetic disaccharide called lactulose. It is made of fructose and galactose. We do not have an enzyme to break this down, therefore it will sit in the intestine and feed the bacteria that are there. This is what produces the gases that are then collect in the test to determine overgrowth or permeability. Lactulose is also used for constipation. We do not have an enzyme to split galactose from fructose, so everyone is lactulose intolerant.

16.2 Lactose Intolerance

There are some cultures that will not carry the genes to produce all disaccharide enzymes. For example, up to 90% of Southern Asians are lactose intolerant.[43] Their bodies are unable to make lactase enzymes. This is not something that can be repaired because the genetic sequences are not able to code for programs that produce these enzymes. This genetics programming is permanent. In these cultures, lactose foods (dairy) are not traditionally an important part of the daily diet. Did these cultures become lactase deficient because of low exposure to milk products following infant weaning, or did the culture avoid dairy products due to intolerance? It's a chicken and egg question really.

Functional lactose intolerance is the inability of a damaged small intestinal cell to produce lactase enzyme properly. This can be repaired over time. It mimics the process that we have previously covered regarding the breakdown of disaccharides. Lactose is made from a galactose plus a glucose molecule. Lactase enzymes are produced in the small intestinal cells. Lactase enzymes are also available in GI Janel Digest C and GI Janel Digest B formulas to aid in the breakdown of lactose and support the tolerance to dairy products.

16.3 SULFUR INTOLERANCE AND DEFICIENCY

Sulfur Intolerance is not the same thing as a sulfa drug allergy or a sulfite intolerance (see chapter on forms of sulfur). Sulfur is an essential element used in the body for building tissues via the important disulfide bond. The disulfide bond literally holds you together, so without sulfur, you would fall apart like a wobbly bowl of jelly. Sulfur is also essential for detoxification (making a toxic molecule less harmful and getting rid of it through the bowels or urine). There are twenty standard amino acids and two of them contain sulfur: methionine and cysteine. You could not survive without sulfur, and it is impossible to be allergic to sulfur. Homocysteine, taurine and cysteine also contain sulfur.

While not completely understood, there are many theories regarding the issue of sulfur intolerance. Like many physiological conditions, there are likely several reasons for sulfur intolerance that act separately or in concert.

Sulfur intolerance is seen in people who do not tolerate the addition of high dietary sulfur and have systemic symptoms when exposed. For these individuals, the sulfur sensitivity can mimic the symptoms of a histamine reaction, with hives, brain fog, flushing, fatigue, nausea, headaches or asthma symptoms.

If a patient has fixed or genetic pathway error causing sulfur intolerance (this is rare), then it is unlikely that the GI Janel One protocol will be an appropriate treatment avenue. However, in my clinical experience, most of those people who notice intolerance symptoms when initiating GI Janel One can eventually tolerate the supplements very well once they've gotten to the higher doses. It simply requires patience and some coaching. Eventually, as the sulfur stores are replenished in the body, histamine symptoms disappear and the therapeutic effects of GI Janel One at higher doses can be achieved very profoundly.

Here is an example of a sulfur intolerant patient using GI Janel One to replenish sulfur stores. I first saw this 50-year-old woman in 2014. She had done many Candida cleanses that helped her, but the symptoms always returned afterwards. I suspected that there may also be some degree of SIBO, and I questioned the strength of her gastrointestinal barrier. She was unwilling to pay for SIBO testing but agreed to treat empirically. She reported gassiness and borborygmus (stomach grumbles). She said that she had incomplete evacuation with bowel movements, gas pain and a constant feeling of bruising and aching in her abdomen. She also told me that she had taken over ten years of daily antibiotics for acne, which she was no longer using. She had a history of testing positive for Candida in her stools, episodes of vaginal yeast and brain fog. She was very reluctant to try GI Janel One as anything new was difficult for her. She agreed to try a tiny pinch of a dose, along with GI Janel Digest B and a soft food diet. She brought me her IgG food testing from years past which showed that she needed to avoid yeast, wheat, corn, tomato, soy, egg and coffee.

When we met two weeks later, she told me that even on the pinch dose of GI Janel One, she noticed an improvement in her borborygmus and gas symptoms, so she was encouraged. However, she also noticed a sensation of her tongue burning along with vaginal burning and itching. She had some natural suppositories at home that she wanted to use for the vaginal symptoms, which resolved this infection nicely. Since I've seen these same symptoms at low doses in other patients who are sulfur intolerant, I asked her to increase to two pinches of GI Janel One, knowing that eventually the unwanted symptoms would stop. When she reached ¼ teaspoon dose of GI Janel One, an old symptom of mouth ulcers began in conjunction with an upper body rash and a flushing feeling, so we kept her at that dose until they cleared. These are also symptoms I've seen in others who believe they are sulfur intolerant. Since these symptoms resolve in the course of the protocol, I believe they are part of the microbiome shifting and will pass. I also suspect that gently coaxing the sulfur pathways in the body upregulates any genetic polymorphisms so that sulfur is handled better. She noted at this time that her acne was much better. By the time she got to ¾ of a teaspoon of GI Janel One, she began to turn a corner. Her allergies and moods were improving. She would have episodes of gurgles and gas following her dose, but not at other times of the day. I assured her this was normal and to continue her pinch dose increases. It took over two years for her to reach the full dose of two tablespoons of GI Janel One. Over this time, her digestive symptoms continued to improve until they were resolved, including those that occurred just after taking her dose of GI Janel One. She began adding foods back into her diet and can now tolerate legumes, corn, tomato, wheat and eggs without symptoms. Her bowels are regular, her skin is clear and there has been no oral ulcer, rash or burning symptoms for years.

I strongly suspect that sulfur intolerance is a compensation for sulfur deficiency. As we've examined previously, digestive sulfur intolerance may be more linked to the shifting microbiome as hydrogen sulfide species are released from the body once the sulfur stores are replenished. This is likely the mechanism behind the initial GI symptoms when using low doses of GI Janel One. I suspect the shift in the microbiome is what leads to the eventual tolerance and benefit at high doses. I have seen this occur hundreds of times in my practice. Taking GI Janel One can cause additional gas that passes (not trapped gas) at the lower doses. Once the IBS/SIBO patient reaches the higher doses and the sulfur stores are replenished, the gas is resolved (typically permanently).

Overgrowth of certain bacteria found in the intestine can contribute to sulfur-based symptoms. These species include Streptococcus, Enterococcus and Prevotella which will use sulfur to make hydrogen sulfide and give a rotten egg smell to your flatulence. Some patients experience their IBS/SIBO as a burning feeling throughout their digestion due to the production of hydrogen sulfide. This can be a very severe symptom. Since GI Janel One is formulated to resolve dysbiosis, as you increase your dose you will be lowering the population of these species and experience this symptom much less, and eventually not at all. I have seen the resolution of this very uncomfortable and mysterious symptom in many patients, often very quickly.

There is an interesting theory proposed by Dr. Greg Nigh, ND, regarding sulfur intolerance. He hypothesizes that SIBO is an adaptive process by the body which occurs when the sulfur metabolic pathways are interfered with and blocked by toxic exposures. He believes that the primary culprit of this interference is the use of pesticides, primarily glyphosate (Round Up). Glyphosate is ubiquitous now. Even people who eat only organic food will have this pesticide stored in their bodies. In fact, all US babies are now born with levels of this pesticide in their bodies. Dr. Nigh theorizes that since the body is unable to produce its own sulfate from dietary sulfur, there is increased growth of sulfur-reducing bacteria in the gut to compensate. This sulfur bacteria then provide the vital sulfur to the body in a usable form. In doing so, these sulfur bacteria also produce a lot of gas in the form of hydrogen sulfide (SIBO).[44]

It is reasoned that this interference by glyphosate inhibits sulfate levels via the chelation of minerals needed for sulfate production, by the interference of sulfur cycle amino acids and by cofactor displacement (molybdenum). The increase of sulfur reducing bacteria then causes higher levels of H2S (hydrogen sulfide) and sulfite (SO3), which can then be directly oxidized into sulfate (SO4). Mitochondria in disseminated cells will oxidize these into the biologically-active sulfur in the form of Paps 3'-Phosphoadenosine-5'-phosphosulfate for use in the body.

Dr. Nigh's treatment plan is to restrict dietary sulfur. He recommends the intake of essential sulfur through the skin using Epsom salt baths (4 cups per bath) daily, which has been determined to increase serum sulfate levels in the body.

Dr. Nigh's results, which sound very impressive, really got me noodling over what might be going on here. How is it that restriction of sulfur gives the same impressive symptom relief from IBS/SIBO symptoms as supplementing sulfur levels? Then I started thinking about one of his other theories. He believes that SIBO and the production of methane and hydrogen gas by bacteria and other species are downstream from the overgrowth of sulfur reducing bacteria. He believes this is because, with a restrictive sulfur diet, the symptoms of methane and hydrogen gas production resolve. But the symptoms of methane and hydrogen gas production also resolve with GI Janel treatment by the addition of sulfur! How do we reason this one out?

Here's what I think is happening. I think that providing adequate levels of sulfur to the body stops the compensation mechanism in the gut that is overgrowing sulfur-fixing microbes. When the body has the sulfur it needs, there is no longer a requirement for the additional sulfur gas-producing bacteria to overgrow. So, these hydrogen sulfide producing bacteria die off and the microbiome distribution of the large and small intestine both benefit. The downstream growth of methane and hydrogen gas-producing species is then eradicated because of the removal of sulfur species as the microbiome balances. There may be more to it than this, but it's my current working theory.

I want to now explore other possibilities of sulfur intolerance. The cause of sulfur sensitivity may be genetic, or it may be due to an upregulation of the detoxification process. When more sulfur is available for the glucuronidation phase II liver detox pathways, you will use the pathway more efficiently. Thus, your body will be detoxifying more rapidly. Glucuronidation is used to remove mineralocorticoids, glucocorticoids, drugs, pollutants, hormones, retinoids and fatty acid derivatives from the body. The pathway prepares these substances for excretion in the stool.

A genetic problem with sulfur metabolism can occur with CBS (Cystathione beta synthase) enzyme defects. The CBS enzyme recycles sulfur and releases ammonia in the recycling process.

The CBS mutations up-regulate or increase the activity of the CBS enzyme. Thus, if you are feeding it more sulfur, there is a potential of more release of ammonia. Excess ammonia can potentially create symptoms of fatigue, nausea, back pain, abdominal pain or confusion.

For people with the CBS defect (this can be tested in saliva with online genetic methylation profiles), I usually prescribe GI Janel One in a more gradual, low-dose, long term schedule to mitigate any adverse effects. It still works, it just takes longer. Dark, leafy greens like kale, collard or spinach contain chlorophyll which can help to neutralize ammonia, can be helpful for patients with the CBS mutations in order to handle sulfur.

Sulfur in the thiol form (when sulfur takes the place of oxygen in the hydroxyl group of an alcohol) can chelate heavy metals. There is the potential for people who have heavy metal toxicity in their bodies to also have symptoms of fatigue and fogginess while using GI Janel One or Core. If metal toxicity is suspected, then I would recommend doing a urinary test for metals following a chelation exposure. (This can be run through a standard lab.)

Glutathione pathways can also be tested with simple genetic testing. I have found many patients who lack efficient glutathione conjugation pathways in their livers. Some of them are very sensitive to the addition of this supplement.

Molybdenum is a cofactor for the enzyme sulfite oxidase which eliminates sulfur from the body. This may be helpful to take with GI Janel One. There are functional labs which can evaluate molybdenum deficiencies. People severely deficient in molybdenum have poorly functioning sulfite oxidase and are prone to reactions to sulfites in foods.

If there is a concern with the body's ability to process sulfur, it makes the most sense to do a 24-hour urine collection for sulfur excretion. This can be done through a standard lab or through a specialty lab as part of a panel. As you proceed in your treatment with the GI Janel One, your body can retain and utilize more of the nutrient, rather than excreting it through the kidneys or bowels. This is another reason for a slow increase in dosing. Urinary sulfate testing has not been approved by the FDA. There can be a range of results based on intake. Therefore, if I use this test, it will be prior to the use of GI Janel One, or I will have the patient stop their dosing for a washout period of two weeks before the urine collection. This test will then reflect the sulfur metabolism and excretion in the urine from the daily protein consumption. [45]

Dysfunctional sulfoxidation pathways are another potential contributor to sulfur intolerance. These pathways are the primary source of inorganic sulfate in the body. If the pathways are not functioning well, protein-rich foods containing cysteine will be slowed or blocked and will not be converted well into inorganic sulfate. This results in an elevation of cysteine or sulfite and a decrease in inorganic sulfate. People with a dysfunctional sulfoxidation pathway may see a worsening of their symptoms with the use of cysteine, methionine or glutathione supplementation due to the potential increase in the cysteine load.[46] If this is a fixed condition, then sulfur may cause an irritation that is ongoing. If this condition can be upregulated by the GI Janel protocol then eventually, sulfur will be more tolerated.

16.4 Forms of Sulfur

16.4.1 Sulfa Drugs (Sulfonamides)

Allergies to sulfa-containing drugs are quite common. Sulfa drugs contain a molecule called sulfonamide. Sulfonamides contain sulfur, oxygen, nitrogen, and hydrogen. The sulfonamide drugs were the first antimicrobial drugs in use (antibiotic.) They stop the bacteria's ability to reproduce. Below is a summary of sulfonamide containing drugs. [47]

Sulfonamide Antibiotics	Thiazide Diuretics	Loop Diuretics	Sulfonylureas	Carbonic Anhydrase Inhibitors
sulfadiazine	hydrochlorothiazide	furosemide	chlorpropamide	
sulfamethoxazole	chlorthiazide		tolbutamide	
sulfasalazine	metolazone		tolazamide	
sulfisoxazole	chlorthalidone		glipizide	
sulfacetamide	indapamide		glyburide	
sulfanilamide	methyclothiazide			
sulfathiazole				
sulfabenzamide				

When a sulfonamide molecule is metabolized in the body, it can attach to proteins and form a larger molecule that can become an allergic antigen. This protein complex is what initiates an allergic response.

Allergic reactions to sulfonamides are serious, and these drugs must be avoided if an allergy is present. Sulfonamides contain sulfur, but the allergy occurs due to the entire sulfonamide molecule, not to the sulfur on its own.

16.4.2 Sulfites

Sulfites are naturally occurring, sulfur-containing molecules that form in the fermentation process. Sulfites (SO3) contain one sulfur atom surrounded by three oxygen atoms. Sulfates (SO4) contain one sulfur atom surrounded by four oxygen atoms. They are a gaseous form of sulfur. When sulfur gas is surrounded by two oxygen atoms (SO2), it is called sulfur dioxide.

Sulfites are used as a preservative in foods. They occur naturally in the process of making beer and wine. Some wine manufacturers add additional sulfites as preservatives. Sulfites have antibacterial and antioxidant properties and are generally considered harmless, except for people who do not have the proper enzymes or cofactors (molybdenum) to convert them. The enzyme required is called sulfite oxidase. The sulfite oxidase enzyme is an intercellular enzyme found in the mitochondria, which is the cellular energy center.

Those who have difficulty converting sulfite to sulfate have a sulfite intolerance. Molybdenum is a required cofactor in this conversion. Sulfite allergies can range from skin rashes, headaches, swelling of mouth or lips, wheezing or allergic symptoms such as rhinitis, asthma, and rarely anaphylaxis. However, sulfite intolerance does not employ classic allergy pathways and is suspected to be more of an intolerance that an allergy. The mechanisms of the reaction are thought to be a cholinergic reflex response, an IgE mediated delayed hypersensitivity or a sulfite oxidase deficiency.[48]

It should be noted that true, genetic sulfite oxidase deficiency is serious and will commonly show up in neonates who are exhibiting symptoms of seizures, dysmorphic features and slow mental development. This is a rare condition with only 50 cases reported worldwide. In most cases, true sulfite oxidase deficiency is fatal in infancy or early childhood.

Approximately 1 in 100 people have sulfite reactions. Their reaction can range from mild to life-threatening.

Examples of foods that may contain sulfites include:

- Baked goods
- Soup mixes
- Jams
- Canned vegetables
- Pickled foods
- Gravies

- Dried fruit
- Potato chips
- Trail mix
- Beer and wine
- Vegetable juices
- Sparkling grape juice
- Apple cider
- Bottled lemon juice and lime juice
- Tea
- Many condiments
- Molasses
- Fresh or frozen shrimp
- Guacamole
- Maraschino cherries
- Dehydrated, pre-cut, or peeled potatoes

Ingredients to look for on food labels include: Sulfur dioxide, potassium bisulfite or potassium metabisulfite, sodium bisulfite, sodium metabisulfite, or sodium sulfite.

If you're sensitive to sulfites, you need to avoid them. It is important that you check labels on all food packages. When you eat out, ask your chef or server if sulfites are used or added to food before or during preparation.[49]

Sulfites are not the same as sulfa drugs. Cross-reactive hypersensitivity between sulfonamide and sulfites is unlikely. Sulfites are not the same as elemental sulfur. Metabolism of elemental sulfur in the intestine is done by bacteria. These bacteria are anaerobic chemoorganotrophs, more specifically, the sulfur- and sulfate- reducing bacteria. These bacteria reduce sulfur to hydrogen sulfide, they do not oxidize sulfur to sulfite.[50]

16.4.3 Sulfates

Sulfates (SO4) contain one sulfur atom surrounded by four oxygen atoms. Sulfates are very important molecules for everyone's health and do not cause allergic or sensitivity reactions. Sulfates are used as escort molecules for several supplements including glucosamine sulfate and vanadyl sulfate. Sulfates are not the same as sulfites and sulfa drugs. Thus, people who are sensitive to sulfites and sulfa drugs are not by extrapolation, sensitive to sulfates.

The production of sulfates occurs in the body when the sulfite oxidase enzyme converts sulfites to sulfates.

Sulfur dioxide (SO2) can cause an irritant reaction in some people, usually asthmatics or highly-allergic individuals. Sulfites (SO3) may trigger asthma, hives, rash, sneezing, swollen or scratchy throat, stomach pain, nausea or diarrhea. Sulfate causes no adverse reaction. It is a natural by-product of metabolism which is excreted in urine.[51]

16.4.4   Sulfur

Sulfur is the chemical element that is found in sulfa drugs, sulfites, and sulfates. Sulfur is an essential element of life. It is a component of amino acids and other important molecules that build the body structure. Sulfur is necessary for the disulfide bonds that literally hold our tissues together. It is *impossible* to have a sulfur allergy. You cannot survive without sulfur. When people say that they are allergic or intolerant to sulfur they mean sulfites or sulfonamide drugs, not to sulfur or sulfates.

Sulfur in GI Janel One is in the form of methylsulfonylmethane (MSM). This is an organosulfur compound with the formula: 2(CH3) SO2. When we have sulfur in our diets or as a supplement, we are introducing it into the anaerobic environment of the intestines. In an anaerobic environment, bacteria and yeast use elemental sulfur or sulfate as the final receptor in the electron transport chain that ultimately provides them with energy. Microbes ferment the products of carbohydrates called pyruvate. Either sulfate or sulfur acts as the electron receptors in the final step of this process.[52]

Sulfur-containing nutrients include alpha-lipoic acid, methyl-sulfonyl-methane (MSM), allicin (the sulfur compound that is the main active ingredient of garlic), glucosamine sulfate, chondroitin sulfate, SAMe (S-adenosylmethionine), and several important antioxidants, such as glutathione, N-acetylcysteine (NAC) and dimethyl-sulfoxide (DMSO).

According to Dr. Stanley W Jacob. MD, in *A Comprehensive Review of the Science and Therapeutics of Methylsulfonylmethane*, "No allergic reactions to MSM have been documented, even though hundreds of our patients with allergies to sulfonamides and to sulfites have taken MSM daily over prolonged periods without incident. Moreover, the only clinical trial of oral MSM to be published in a peer-reviewed scientific journal utilized the compound as a treatment for seasonal allergies. There is currently no evidence to support the concern that MSM supplementation could trigger reactions arising from sulfonamide allergy or sulfite insensitivity."[53]

16.5 HISTAMINE INTOLERANCE

Histamine is naturally occurring in foods such as aged meats, tofu, champagne, eggplant, canned meat and fish, and spinach. More histamine food list can be found online. This large list of foods can be extensive and overwhelming. The good news is that once treatment with GI Janel supports and repairs the integrity of the gastrointestinal barrier, histamine intolerance improves.

Histamine intolerance is a bit of a buzz word right now. Like a lot of GI issues, the intolerance is a symptom of gastrointestinal barrier weakness. Resolve the gastrointestinal barrier and microbiome issues and histamine intolerance resolves too.

Histamine intolerance can mimic the bloating and cramping of IBS/SIBO, so if symptoms continue while on your supplements, even with the level one soft food diet, then take out histamine foods until you are stronger. In 20 years, I have never needed to put anyone on a low histamine diet to resolve their IBS/SIBO symptoms.

In my clinic, we use desensitization to lower overall histamine reactions, and speed up the recovery from histamine hypersensitivity. We also use IV nutrients that support the histamine degradation process so that histamine is broken down more efficiently. Mycotoxin load from mold can also contribute to histamine intolerance and to mast cell activation syndrome. This occurs as the mycotoxins shift the TH1 (T helper cell) and TH2 cell balance. If mycotoxins are detected in the body, removing them is imperative. These are detected with a urine test offered through a functional laboratory.

16.6 OXALATE INTOLERANCE

Oxalates are most well known in their calcium oxalate form in kidney stones. They occur in plant foods like leafy greens. High oxalate content foods may also irritate the GI lining in the preliminary stages of recovery so if they are a problem, reserve them for addition gradually after you have completed your GI Janel protocol. Possible abdominal symptoms include pain, bloating, constipation, diarrhea, gas, indigestion and heartburn.

High oxalate foods include beans, beer, beets, berries, chocolate, coffee, cranberries, spinach, nuts, oranges, rhubarb, cola, soy beans, sweet potatoes and tofu. More extensive lists can be found online.[54] These foods can mimic the symptoms of IBS/SIBO, so if symptoms continue while on your supplements even with the level one soft food diet, then take out high oxalate foods until you are stronger.

16.7 SALICYLATE INTOLERANCE

In plants, salicylates are part of the natural protection against diseases, insects, fungal growth and bacteria.

Salicylates are the salts and esters of salicylic acid. This is an organic acid that is a key ingredient in aspirin and other pain medications and is frequently found in cosmetics and beauty products.

These can cause many systemic symptoms for people with a sensitivity to them. The gastrointestinal symptoms are nausea, stomach pain and diarrhea. We know that salicylate intolerance can be improved using omega three oils and other anti-inflammatories, and can improve with the GI Janel protocol, which strengthens the digestive system. I am never a fan of removing whole, healthy foods from the diet, so the sooner resolution can occur and the sooner the system becomes strengthened, the sooner a whole food diet can be resumed.

Foods that are high in salicylates include dried fruit, berries, apricot, avocado, dates, grapes, oranges, green olives, nightshades (eggplant, potato, peppers, tomato), almonds, coconut, olive oil and honey.

These foods can mimic the symptoms of IBS/SIBO, so if symptoms continue while on your supplements and the level one soft food diet, then take out high salicylate foods until you are stronger.

16.8 MAST CELL ACTIVATION SYNDROME

Historically, mast cell activation syndrome (MCAS) was reserved for rare genetic defects that affected only a very small portion of the population. In 2010 the disorder was renamed idiopathic mast cell activation syndrome. This is a clinical diagnosis once genetic defects have been ruled out. Idiopathic means that the cause is unknown.

Allergies are caused by the release of histamines from mast cells (in addition to hundreds of other cytokines and chemical messengers). The mast cell is over 500,000,000 years old and is the original neuro-immunological cell.

Gastrointestinal symptoms of this syndrome may respond well to antihistamine therapies. The digestive symptoms include pain, cramping, nausea, vomiting, diarrhea, and heartburn (reflux). The heartburn may be increased by the increased release of gastric acid from parietal cells in the stomach when they are stimulated by the histamines. Once again, I believe this syndrome to be a symptom of the health of the gastrointestinal barrier rather than a stand-alone diagnosis.

Idiopathic means "we don't know why this happens." In mast cell activation syndromes this confusion is compounded by the fact that foods seem to cause intermittent reactions, so it is difficult to pin down when and what the issue is.

Since this is a histamine-based reaction to a variety of foods, in my clinic we treat this with allergy desensitization treatments. We see profound resolution of symptoms for patients who have a wide variety of histamine based (allergy) reactions in the digestive system. This provides patients with an alternative treatment to ongoing suppressive therapies with cromolyn sodium, antihistamines and anti-leukotrienes.

There is also strong evidence linking MCAS and histamine intolerance to mold toxicity. Tests are now available to detect mold or mycotoxins in the body. These have become very helpful when looking for a cause for these mysterious symptoms.

16.9 CANDIDA

There is not a lot to say about this diagnosis that I haven't covered elsewhere. Candida overgrowth in the small intestine is SIFO. Candida overgrowth in the large intestine is part of the large intestinal dysbiosis syndrome and is also referred to as LIFO (Large Intestinal Fungal Overgrowth). Candida represents 90% of the fungal species in the small intestine and the majority in the large intestine. When these fungal species overgrow, they use the food you eat to create a gassy pain and bloating that is like bacterial overgrowth symptoms. Remember, if you have gassy symptoms, it is bacteria or fungal species using your food to make gas. You cannot make the gas yourself. Candida overgrowth can occur in the small intestine, large intestine or both, and it can grow independently of bacterial overgrowth or with it. When I see patients, who have undergone SIBO treatments yet continue to have symptoms, I suspect fungal overgrowth or system weakness and regrowth. Candida cannot be tested in the small intestine directly, unless it's done during an endoscopy. This is not a common practice. It can be suspected based on organic acid testing. Sometimes we're lucky enough to get a positive stool test for Candida or another fungal species. Stool testing is a good starting place for baseline diagnostics. Another diagnostic option is to do a clinical trial with an antifungal medication. If symptoms improve, then Candida or another fungal species have been eliminated and the diagnosis can be confirmed.

Here is a very typical case of a recurrent Candida diagnosis in a 48-year-old woman who came in several years ago. When I saw her for her first visit, she complained of six years of digestive symptoms. She said that she had to sleep on the couch in order to be close to the bathroom, and she was exhausted by sleep that was interrupted by digestive pain and diarrhea. Initially she had been diagnosed with reflux and put on acid blockers. This made her symptoms worse because acidity is necessary to keep yeast from overgrowing in the small intestine (SIFO). Her gastroenterologist performed an endoscopy, colonoscopy and blood work, and gave her a diagnosis of gastritis (inflammation in the stomach). She then saw an ND who diagnosed her with Candida and put her on some natural antifungals. Her symptoms resolved on this treatment. Two months later, when she was under a great deal of family stress, all her symptoms came back worse than ever. The reason that her symptoms returned is the same reason that SIBO symptoms return. If the body does not get the raw nutrients it needs to heal and strengthen, or if it is overwhelmed by inflammatory reactions to food, the overgrowth can return. This was exactly what happened for this patient. When the symptoms returned, she went back to her gastroenterologist who repeated her colonoscopy and endoscopy, found gastritis still present and put her on Zantac (acid blocker). When I saw her after this, she complained of abdominal pain, loose stools and severe weight loss due to pain on eating. Her weight was at 94 pounds. I attempted to wean her off a myriad of supplements and focus on digestion at her first visit. I started her on GI Jan-Aloe, collected blood for IgG antibodies to food and for celiac disease, and had her collect a stool sample for a fungal culture.

When she returned four weeks later, she told me that her abdominal pain had improved, but she occasionally had a sharp pain in her lower abdomen. She said that she was having a lot of gas and was only able to eat chicken and gluten free noodles. Her stool test was positive for Candida glabrata and her celiac HLA was positive for one genetic variant. Her IgG was positive for whole eggs, yeast and sugar. I kept her off these foods and asked her to do a soft food diet. I had her take a two-week course of voriconazole as an antifungal and return in four weeks. After this treatment her stools turned from loose diarrhea to constipation which responded well to over-the-counter fiber supplements. I had her add in an evening dose of GI Janel AM/BM to help keep her bowels moving so the remaining yeast would not overgrow in the stagnation.

After being on the GI Jan-Aloe, her gastritis had resolved enough that we were able to start her on GI Janel Digest C formula and GI Janel One. I had her start with 1/16 of a teaspoon a day. When she returned, she told me that the One formula initially gave her a rash on her neck (Herx) followed by a clearing of that rash and of her rosacea rash on her face. She continued to very slowly increase her GI Janel One formula to the full dose of 2 tablespoons per day over the course of many months. During that time, she expanded her diet and was able to gain back her weight to 113 pounds. She no longer needed to sleep on the couch close to the restroom, and reported no reflux, no abdominal pain, and no gassiness or bloating.

17 TESTS

17.1 IGG SERUM TESTS

Serum IgG testing through a specialty lab has been one of the most helpful methods in determining foods that adversely affect digestion. IgG is an antibody, and antibodies are made by the immune system in response to bacteria, viruses, fungus, animal dander or cancer cells. You can think about it this way: antibodies attach to foreign substances and "tag" them, so the immune system can find and destroy them. Antibodies are extremely specific to their target.

There are four main antibodies that we produce in our immune system.

IgG – can be cytotoxic, immune complexed or even associated with delayed hypersensitivity when the T cells become involved.

IgE – are immediate antibody reactions and are involved in allergy and anaphylactic reactions.

IgA – are in the tubular systems of the body (the lungs and digestive system). They protect us from foreign invasions there.

IgM – are early onset antibody reactions (the first antibody that is released to handle infections). For example, when you first contract the mononucleosis virus called Epstein-Barr, the initial protective antibody to appear is the IgM form. This is tested with the EBV monospot test.

IgG antibody reactions can range from immediate to delayed (if the T cells become involved in the inflammatory process). Because of this, you may not realize which food is the problem. Consider for example that you eat scrambled eggs every day for breakfast, but your symptoms are delayed and do not occur until several hours later or the next day. In this case, it's difficult to correlate your symptoms to the egg exposure. Or, say you eat a lot of sugar on Monday and Wednesday and by Thursday you are bloated in pain. This can be the result of the accumulation of your diet's impact, compounded by a delayed reaction. It would be difficult to determine that sugar from days ago was the cause of your symptoms.

These blood tests usually cost under $200 and analyze close to 100 foods. I have listed my preferred lab in the index. An alternative to this test is food elimination. Foods that adversely affect the digestive system are dairy, gluten, wheat, whole eggs, sugar, soy, yeasts and sometimes corn. By taking these foods out of your diet and using a soft food diet, you may avoid IgG testing.

Some other alternative food testing methods are available, which look for inflammatory responses to foods. I have not found these to be accurate for digestive symptoms.

There are also some IgG tests available through standard labs. The standard labs employ a different testing method and tend to show all foods as positives; thus, they are not very helpful. Additionally, they charge more than $50 per food, so this adds up quickly. IgG testing is typically seen as investigational by insurance, so you may end up paying the bill in the long run when going through a standard lab.

17.1.1 Interpreting IgG tests

Now that I've told you about the benefits of IgG testing, let me tell you about its downfalls. Mainly, there can be (not always) false positives that show up on the test results. Therefore, I pay attention to two factors on these panels.

If a food is positive and is in the list of foods that adversely affect the digestive system (dairy, wheat, gluten, whole eggs, yeast, sugar, soy and perhaps corn), then remove this food from your diet.

If you have other reactions, for example, to cranberry or banana, this may be a false positive (reads positive on the test but is not affecting your digestive symptoms). Unless you know that these potentially false positive foods impact your digestive symptoms, you need not avoid them.

These false positives may also be a sign of leaky gut. For some people, chronic inflammation has damaged the gastrointestinal barrier enough so that all food can be in contact with the immune system. In this case, antibodies are formed to all foods and the panel results show low to moderate reactivity to every food tested. This is the second thing I pay attention to with this testing method. The treatment remains the same though: remove the food(s) from the list above so they stop irritating your digestive system. The other foods that are positive will have a reduction in inflammatory production once the main trigger foods are out of the diet.

This test is certainly not 100% accurate, but it is the best that is commercially available so far to correlate mysterious GI symptoms to food interference. It has proven accurate in identifying problem foods for about 90% of my digestive patients.

17.1.2 IgG stages of healing

Once you know what foods you react to, you have gained powerful information that you can use to begin feeling remarkably better. You can put aside difficult diets and start to treat and resolve your specific food intolerances.

When using your IgG results, there are three main phases of healing. If you follow these directions, you will be able to understand where you are in the process of healing your digestive food intolerance. Remember, these IgG results are not a life sentence. You will not have to avoid the identified foods forever. IgG results are a guideline to healing the gastrointestinal barrier by removing the irritation caused by the food and allowing the system to strengthen. They are rarely a permanent, lifetime concern.

Throughout this process of recovery, take your digestive supplements with your food, as these will assist in decreasing irritation and healing the gastrointestinal barrier.

In my clinic, we use immunotherapy treatment to expedite this process of food elimination and decrease the time needed to avoid the foods. We desensitize for tolerance, so that the immune system can more quickly stop its unnecessary attack on foods. This option speeds up the food elimination phases considerably for my patients.

17.1.2.1 *Healing Phase One: Hyper reactive. (12 months)*

Imagine your immune cells have been creating antibodies to protect you against a food for months or years. What a lot of unnecessary work this is for your immune system.

If you take the food out of your diet, what happens to all those cells that are prepared to release inflammatory chemicals when they see the food? They are stockpiling those histamine and cytokine chemicals.

The white blood cells which in the past were working so hard to create inflammation are now resting and stocking their chemicals. They are ready for when or if the food arrives in their path again. This means that if you've completely removed the food like cow dairy products out of your diet, the cells are ready and waiting to protect you when that food arrives again, and the forces to respond are stronger than ever.

I've seen the following scenario many times in practice and have experienced it myself. A patient will avoid the food for a couple of weeks and symptoms will abate nicely. Then they may have some of the food either accidentally or on purpose. This is when we can really appreciate the power of our food and our immune system. Symptoms that have been decreasing, like abdominal pain, diarrhea, gas, nausea and vomiting, can be immediate and severe with an exposure following elimination in phase one.

I like this analogy: if you throw a rock into choppy, turbulent water, it is difficult to see the effect of its impact. If you throw a rock into still water, the effect is obvious. Once you've avoided the foods, your inflammation calms down and you become more like the still water.

This first stage lasts for roughly twelve to twenty-four months for foods that you will eventually be able to eat freely again. The first stage passes much more quickly for children than for adults. Children may be able to re-introduce foods in less than twelve months.

As you go through the stages of this process, you will determine the foods that will eventually not be a problem for you versus those you'll need to limit or avoid long term. The good news is that there will only be one or two of these if you have done the treatments that will support the healing of your digestion.

Twelve months, you say! She wants me to not eat gluten or dairy for twelve to twenty-four months?

Yes, I do. It's part of your healing process, and it's worth it. If you feel discouraged, read ahead to the next phase for comfort. Also, desensitization is available to speed up this process.

> Here's a case to keep you inspired. I first saw this 25-year old patient in 2012. She came in with IgG testing from another clinic, but it was not the one I typically use and showed reactions to foods that do not tend to have an adverse effect on digestion. She had taken the indicated foods out of her diet with no change in her digestive symptoms. She reported feeling gassy and bloated with painful distention of her stomach. She was also constipated and had a bowel movement every three days. I began her on GI Janel Digest B formula and AM/BM formula to regulate her bowels. She agreed to repeat her IgG tests with the lab I prefer and was found positive for cow dairy and gluten. We removed these from her diet and added back: basil, beef, black pepper, cantaloupe, cauliflower, cinnamon, cocoa, crab, ginger, green beans, kale, lobster, mushroom, mustard, oats, peanut, spinach, squash, tarragon and brewer's yeast, which had been removed based on the previous testing. She returned four weeks later and told me that her digestive symptoms were improving and so were her muscle aches and fatigue. At this point we moved to desensitization for the gluten and dairy at eight-week intervals. Six months later she reported to me that she had eaten regular pizza with gluten and cheese and had no

symptoms from this. She had determined that if she does not consume pizza more than three times a week, she has no symptoms of bloating, gas or constipation. If she has too much cheese and gluten, she will have these symptoms, but they will resolve in a few hours.

Children can challenge foods for re-introduction earlier because their bodies are more able to adapt to changes and they typically have a stronger healing capacity (vital force).

For adults, the long-term digestive symptoms take a toll over time on the rest of the body, taxing the nervous system, immune system and endocrine system. Therefore, the recovery from food-based symptoms is less expedient than for children.

One helpful prescription for people who do not want to be strict with their diet is the addition of cromolyn sodium, also called Gastrochrom. This can be taken in 200 mg doses, 15 minutes before eating, so that the body is less reactive to food intolerances.

17.1.2.2 Phase Two: Healing and challenge

The road to recovery! You've just finished the most challenging part of your journey, which is where you must eliminate irritating foods.

Now that your immune cells have not seen their enemy food for months, the troops begin to retreat. Those white blood cells that have been misinformed to protect you from foods now travel to storage tissues where they are no longer immediately available to react.

Not only that, but because the chronic inflammatory response to food has ended, those cells of the intestinal tube can now seal back up (given the right support) with their tight junctions and their strong basement membrane and become the highly selective transport system they were meant to be. You have repaired the gastrointestinal barrier!

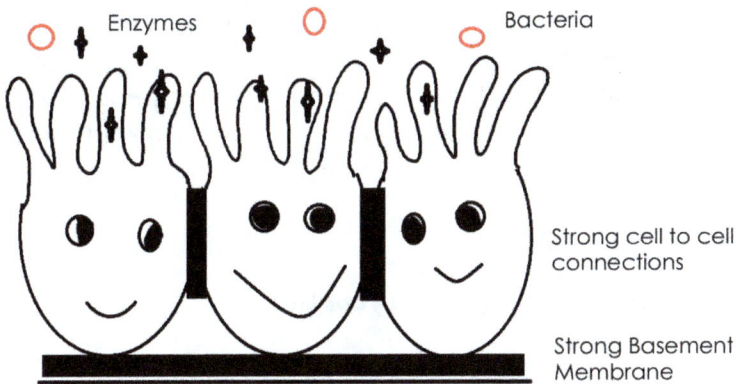

Figure 17.1 A Healthy GI Barrier

At this point, you can begin your food challenge.

Step One – Have a little bit of the food you have been avoiding (see index for food quantities).

Step Two – WAIT for a minimum of 5 days and observe whether any symptoms return. If they do, you are not ready for that food. Continue to avoid it for another 3- 6 months.

Step Three – If you do not have any return of digestive symptoms, you can begin to eat this food in tiny amounts on a weekly basis (see index for amounts).

Continue with your next food in line to challenge and follow the same procedure. Throughout this process, keep taking your digestive supplements. Your GI Janel digestive formulas will help to break down any potential irritation and will take some stress off digestion. Reserve Dairy and Gluten for your final challenge foods.

In the end, once you've challenged all your foods, you will either have a short list of foods to avoid for another six months or you will be gradually integrating all of the previously problematic foods back into your diet.

By now, you'll know your body well enough to know when you've had too much of something. For example, if you've challenged dairy and gluten successfully, you may decide to order a large pizza and eat most of it. After this, you may not feel so great. This is because there can still be a quantitative response by your body (meaning you overwhelmed it), so be nice to yourself and don't do that.

17.1.2.3 *Phase three: The rest of your life*

Once you've completed your food challenge, you'll be very aware of the foods you can or cannot eat, and you will begin to become aware of the quantity and frequency you can tolerate of the foods that you remain sensitive to.

If you have followed the phases above, you should be able to integrate most foods that were previously problematic back into your diet.

Some people will always have a problem with gluten, but this has more to do with the changes made to the gluten protein than you (see chapter on gluten).

Some people may have congenital or genetically-based lactose intolerance. In this case, lactose-free or low-lactose daily products may be the only type of cow dairy tolerated without symptoms of gas, pain or diarrhea.

In general, choose whole, organic, unprocessed, unrefined foods that are not packaged or made with chemical preservatives. This choice will provide you with more nutrition in order to maintain the health of your whole body.

17.2 Skin Patch Testing

I have begun to use skin patch testing to determine food reaction instead of IgG testing. This has quickly become my test of choice because it will tell us not only if you are responding to a food with delayed antibodies, but if you are responding to a food with any of the hundreds of inflammatory cytokines that are produced in the body. Patch testing is currently only available in my clinic.

17.3 Functional Stool Testing

Another helpful test to run is a functional stool test. This testing is done at a lab which is out of network. (See index.)

In attempting to resolve symptoms, the microbiome is a significant piece of the puzzle. With functional stool tests, you will receive information on how well your body is breaking down the foods you eat, what the status of probiotic growth is in your large intestine, and any infections present in the large intestine (yeast, bacteria, parasites). You can even use these tests to interpret SIBO status.

If the testing is positive for *Methanobrevibacter smithii*, the level of fermentable proteins is high and pancreatic elastase output is low, then it's likely that SIBO is present in the small intestine in addition to what is found in the large intestine stool testing. Of course, you can always confirm this with a direct SIBO breath test.

17.3.1 IBS-D/SIBO

IBS-D/SIBO patients will often have an overgrowth of nonpathogenic bacteria or yeasts in their digestive system. Standard (conventional) lab tests for the stool do not look for these. This is the reason that your stool tests from standard labs come back saying there is nothing wrong.

A standard lab will look for the known pathogenic strains of bacteria, virus and parasites that cause diarrhea. Conventional stool testing is limited to the following species:

- Bacterial cultures: campylobacter, salmonella, shigella
- Toxin testing: clostridium difficile, Escherichia coli
- Ova and parasite testing: parasites, parasite eggs and cysts
- Antigen testing: *Giardia lamblia, Entamoeba histolytica, Cryptosporidium parvum*, rotavirus

Conventional stool tests will not look for chronic growth of nonpathogenic species or potentially pathogenic species of bacteria. Treating people with diarrhea-predominant symptoms based on functional stool results can be very helpful. Those IBS-D/SIBO patients who have symptoms that do not respond to dietary changes can get symptom relief by removing these unwanted bacteria from the body.

I have used herbal antibiotic treatments and prescription antibiotic treatments in these cases. The choice depends on the patient's goals and time frame. We decide together. I provide the options and the patient decides what they would like to do for their symptom resolution. Having said that, most opt for antibiotic treatments along with high probiotic re-seeding. It's much faster and very effective. Using antibiotics in this way, we can control the re-seeding of the beneficial bacteria (microbiome) in the space occupied by the unwanted species that is now freed up by the antibiotics.

Your digestive system is like a bus in rush hour traffic. It will always be full. It is the perfect, dark, warm, moist, anaerobic environment with a steady stream of food coming through for bacterial and yeast growth. If one seat is given up by someone who gets off the bus, another will take its place. Please never use antibiotics without taking an approved probiotic. And please do not take bacterial probiotics that have not been approved by a knowledgeable practitioner. Probiotics are literally bacteria.

Other testing to determine the cause of diarrhea symptoms may include stool testing for pancreatic enzymes, white blood cells, stool fat, lactoferrin, calprotectin or occult blood. Blood tests for diarrhea can test for ASCA antibodies, carcinoid tumor, and celiac antibodies.

> A 57-year-old man who came to see me reported a 30-year history of abdominal pain followed by diarrhea. The pain was relieved after he had an urgent bowel movement. These episodes would occur two to three times a week and he thought that dairy made them worse and more frequent. I started him on GI Janel Digest B formula and a probiotic while we ran tests to rule out celiac disease, inflammatory bowel disease and an IgG panel. His results came back normal and his IgG panel showed only a very mild elevation to dairy and sugar. I requested that he do a 14-day elimination then a five-day challenge of the dairy and sugar and collect stool for a functional digestive panel. He did notice an increase in pain and in diarrhea with the dairy challenge but continued to have symptoms even off dairy.

> The stool test came back with no growth of Lactobacillus and with a Klebsiella bacteria growing in high amounts. It is interesting and very common to see no growth of a probiotic species (Lactobacillus) that he had just been taking in high doses. There is no growth of this because the system is not healthy enough to support its growth. The Klebsiella pneumonia is considered a non-pathogenic species in the digestive system, and therefore is not something that is checked on a regular, conventional panel. However, it is still not a normal stool bacterium and here is a man with symptoms, so it's worth the assumption that for him, this bacterium is an issue. Klebsiella pneumonia is a serious infection if it occurs in the lungs (pneumonia), blood, brain, heart, skin or urinary system. The functional lab does a test for bacterial sensitivity. That means that the lab tests for what will kill the Klebsiella. It was resistant to one antibiotic, but sensitive to five others and we chose to do a fourteen-day course of cephalexin with a daily dose of 200 billion probiotics.

> When he returned to see me, he told me that if he takes his digest B supplement, he now has no pain and no diarrhea regardless of what he eats, including dairy. This means that the problem all along was the Klebsiella

growing in his intestine. Now that it is eliminated, he is free to eat whatever he wants, without symptoms, as long as he is supporting his digestion with the Digest B formula. He was amazed. At his first appointment, he came in saying that he was expecting it to take a long time to resolve this symptom that he had been dealing with for decades, but we cleared it up in a few weeks.

17.3.2   IBS-C/SIBO

Most patients who present with long-term constipation will have some form of yeast overgrowth in their stools. This is because yeasts *love* a warm, dark, quite environment to thrive. SIFO occurs is when this yeast overgrows in the small intestine. SIFO is far more common than what is currently understood. Yeast treatments can be very beneficial for patients with gassy symptoms.

It is typically the patients with chronic constipation who have the greatest variety of unwanted or disruptive bacteria in their test results. I've seen up to ten unwanted species of bacteria and up to three species of yeast testing positive in these results.

If these unwanted bacteria are in the body, then they must be removed for symptoms to be resolved. Sometimes, the body can re-balance itself with the use of supplements and the soft food diet. But more often, we will want to use some herbal or prescriptive medications to help rid the body of these unwanted species. Until the colon has been cleared of the unwanted bacteria and yeast, it will be very difficult to resolve the constipation. Unlike diarrhea-predominant digestive issues, prescription antibiotics are not the best choice here. A slower, more natural treatment will cause fewer side effects and a more lasting resolution of symptoms.

Organic acid profiles may be an option to determine yeast overgrowth. Often the stool testing for yeast comes back negative when it is obvious by the clinical symptoms that yeast is present. The yeast may be a Candida species or one of several other yeast species. Organic acid testing relies on breakdown products of yeast in the body, and if high, it is reasonable to infer that this overgrowth is in the small or large intestine, where there are gassy symptoms.

By far, the most accurate test for SIFO would be a sample taken from the small intestine while performing an endoscopy. This, however, is not typically done.

17.3.3   IBS-M / SIBO (Mixed or Alternating Diarrhea / Constipation)

Cases of mixed or alternating diarrhea and constipation (IBS-M) respond so well to dietary intervention and supplement support that I rarely use functional stool testing in this population. Eliminating, then challenging, and using the GI Janel One protocol will eliminate alternating diarrhea and constipation over time very nicely.

17.4 SIBO TESTS

SIBO testing has fallen off the radar of insurance companies and is currently done in functional medical clinics as an out of pocket expense. I have listed some of the available labs in my index.

SIBO is a breath test. There are many interferences that can occur to invalidate the results of testing, so it is important to prepare yourself and avoid the medications and foods that the lab will specify. Once collected, the sample is mailed to the lab for processing.

You will want to use a lab test that collects samples over the course of 3 or more hours and measures both methane and hydrogen gases. Some labs will also allow additional testing for lactose, glucose and fructose intolerance.

The test measures gases that are created by bacterial fermentation of the challenge substance in your small intestine.

The time that the peak of the gases occurs correlates to the location of the overgrowth in your small intestine. There are up and coming tests that will measure hydrogen sulfide gases in the breath. We look forward to having these available soon.

17.5 LGS Tests

I will typically use the IgG food panel to determine LGS (GI permeability or the overall breakdown in the gastrointestinal barrier). Multiple low-level reactions occurring in a panel are indicative of the presence of LGS.

Functional labs provide a test for Zonulin, which can be measured in the stool. Zonulin is released into the stool when there is damage to the gastrointestinal barrier. When Zonulin is high, there is damage occurring to the tight junctions between the cells of the digestive tract. The tight junction damage allows the interface between the intestinal contents and the immune system and triggers inflammation as a result.

LPS (lipopolysaccharide) endotoxins from gut bacteria are present in endotoxemia, and this correlates to GI permeability. This test is included in the Intestinal Antigenic Permeability Screen (see index). High LPS levels have been correlated to auto-immune diseases, specifically auto-immune thyroid disorders. High LPS may also be related to mysterious diagnoses of leukocytosis (high white blood cell count), low iron levels, blood clotting disorders and thrombocytopenia. By *mysterious* I mean that the reasons have been evaluated and it is still not clear why your body is showing these problems on your lab work.

18 Gluten

18.1 What's up with Gluten?

You might be asking yourself why you're hearing so much about gluten these days. Why is this buzz of gluten free food sweeping the nation? Is it another fad?

Gluten is a protein found in wheat, rye, barley, triticale, spelt, kamut, ferro, durum, bulger and semolina.

There is a very easy way to determine if you have a problem with gluten. Stop eating it for two weeks. Then have some and wait for five days before having anymore. If your body doesn't like gluten, you will know. Use commercial, processed wheat for your challenge food; it will give you the most dramatic effect.

If you are continuously eating gluten, the message gets attenuated and you may not feel great overall, but you won't suspect that gluten as the culprit until you remove it, let your body's inflammation calm down, and then add it back in.

Imagine again a choppy, turbulent lake, all stirred up and moving around. If you throw a rock into that water and you will hardly notice its effect.

If you throw a rock into a still body of water, its impact is obvious. Just try it.

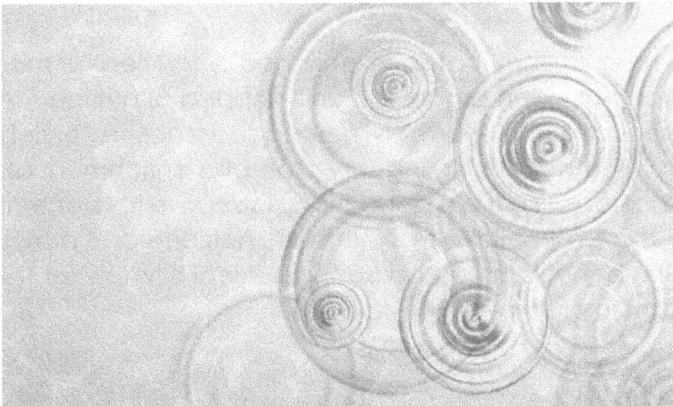

Figure 18.1
Perspective

18.2 ANCIENT WHEAT IS NOT TODAY'S WHEAT

18.2.1 First, Remove the Nutrients

Gluten has been changed over the years. The first change was when we began to remove all the nutrients from the whole wheat grain. The milling process in the 1870's began to strip the bran, oils, and germ out of the grain to make it processed. Most of the nutrients were taken out of the wheat grain to produce the delicious, doughy white flour that we love. It has also been bleached to appear whiter.

White flour is tasty and has a much longer shelf life than whole wheat flour. It ships and stores better to allow for a longer distribution chain.

The nutrients in whole wheat are vitamin E, vitamin K and the B vitamins: thiamin (B1), riboflavin (B2), niacin (B3), folate, pantothenic acid (B5), choline and betaine. Whole wheat contains the minerals calcium, iron, magnesium, phosphorus, potassium, sodium, manganese, selenium and copper. Whole wheat also contains omega-3 and omega-6 fats as well as healthy plant phytosterols.

In contrast, refined and bleached white flour has all vitamins removed except for 25% of the folate. Refined white flour retains the list of minerals; however, the concentration of the minerals is reduced up to 90% of that in whole wheat. This is the same for the omega fats and phytosterols.

When you read a label that says "enriched or fortified," it means that the food has been processed and stripped of nutrients. A synthetic version of the vitamin is then added back to "enrich" the product. The advertising industry promotes enrichment of grains and cereals like it is a good thing. I suppose it's better than nothing, but I don't believe that synthetic nutrients can provide equal health benefits in comparison to nutrient complexes that naturally exist in plants.[55] [56]

18.2.2 Messing with Genetics and new chemicals

The second thing that happened to make gluten more of a problem occurred in the 1960s. At this time, wheat started to be genetically manipulated so that it would yield higher crops. This was done by hybridizing the seeds to create a semi-dwarf wheat. This new wheat, when grown with new fertilizers and pesticides that were manufactured around the same time, enormously increased the crop yield. This was also the beginning of large companies like Dupont and Monsanto becoming fiscally invested in farming technology.

As a result, we now have altered wheat seeds that are grown in synthetic soils and bathed in chemicals. These seeds are then deconstructed, pulverized, bleached and chemically treated to create food. It's hard not to see how this version of wheat might make us feel sick.

18.3 MY HISTORY WITH GLUTEN

Many years ago, I attended a full weekend lecture series entirely on the topic of gluten. I was a young doctor then and was desperate to find some answers that could genuinely address the cause of my patients' health concerns.

The conference speaker looked out at all the physicians in the room and said, "I bet you're going to take this information back to your clinics on Monday morning and tell your patients what to do and what not to do regarding gluten consumption, right?" We all agreed that it was valuable information and we would take it back to our practices on Monday morning, armed with reams of studies and scientific proof to convince our patients of the potential perils of gluten.

Then he asked us, "But how many of you are going to use this information for yourselves?" Well, I certainly wasn't planning on it! I was fine, my digestion was fine at this point and I had energy and my skin was great, thank you very much, but I want my gluten!

Then he challenged us to do two weeks of a gluten free diet. We all agreed that we would eliminate gluten for two full weeks, in the name of research.

It was December and there were lots of festivities during those two weeks, but I kept my promise and avoided gluten completely... until, just under the two-week mark, at a party, without thinking, I grabbed some regular crackers and ate them. It wasn't until later that I realized what I had done, and I felt fine! Yeah, glad that's over.

Here's the part where the five-day challenge (delayed reaction) comes in.

There are delayed reactions to gluten, especially for the "gluten intolerant" people. I spent the rest of the following day sicker than I had ever been.

I have rarely vomited in my life, but that morning spent two solid hours vomiting. There were no signs of any other reason for this, such as an infection. It was clearly the gluten. Since then, if gluten sneaks into my diet, I have the same reaction: a few hours will go by, then my mouth will start to water, and I am running to find a bathroom. This is a fixed intolerance which means it will not resolve with the removal of gluten and the repair of the gastrointestinal barrier. I am motivated to avoid gluten. I have tested negative for celiac biopsy and celiac HLA genetic sequences. I have tested positive to IgG gluten reactions.

I want to emphasize how important the five-day challenge is. Immediate reactions are obvious, but if you have a delayed response, then it may take several days before you begin to have symptoms. If you wait only 24 hours and then become more liberal with your diet, it can be very confusing to determine the cause of your symptoms.

18.4 GLUTEN-INTOLERANCE OPTIONS

If you want to test whether you can tolerate the original form of gluten that existed before wheat grain was hybridized and grown with chemicals, there are companies online that offer ancient grains. More and more these ancient grains are available in stores as well. You may also try spelt grain, which is a close cousin of ancient wheat.

Test these foods to see if you tolerate them. If you do, then it is not the original gluten itself that you are reacting to, it is the changes that have been made to the wheat to increase production and yield. Washington State University is working to develop an ancient grain wheat. At this point, doing a search for ancient grain wheat or heirloom wheat will bring up plenty of options for local or mail order products.[57]

Sourdough bread can be another option for people with either gluten or yeast intolerance. I'm referring to traditional, not commercial, sourdough. Traditional sourdough is made in small batches and has no more than six ingredients. It is made using lactobacillus in combination with gentle yeasts strains. That is the real stuff. Commercial products are mass produced and are found in the regular bread aisles of a grocery.

For some people, the lactobacillus can break down the gluten enough that these breads are better tolerated. In any event, sourdough bread is a healthier choice because the yeast strains are less invasive, and the lactobacillus works well with our digestion. Traditional sourdough, however, does not meet the criteria of less than 20 parts per million gluten, which is required to be classified as gluten free. [58]

There are other grains that replace the products you are accustomed to purchasing. The gluten-free grains are easy to spot on packaging labels. Included are products made from rice, millet, quinoa, corn, buckwheat, oats, sorghum and teff. There are also nuts that can be made into flours for people on paleo diets.

Spelt is an ancient grain relative of wheat and is sometimes classified with common wheat. It has not been manipulated to the same degree as commercial wheat and can be tolerated by some people.

An interesting phenomenon that I have noted is that when my patients travel to Europe and other countries outside of North America, they tolerate the wheat strains and breads there much better. This may be due to the ancient strains, less refining and chemical exposure, enrichment, or all the above. I have hundreds of stories from patients who get dog sick when eating gluten or dairy in North America but tolerate these foods perfectly fine when travelling outside of North America (particularly to Europe). What's the difference? It's the quality of the food itself.

18.5 CELIAC

Celiac disease is a genetically programed inflammatory response to gluten. Unfortunately, once the inflammation becomes active, any exposure to gluten will damage the intestinal cell wall and gastrointestinal barrier. Over time, the intestinal damage leads to malabsorption of nutrients. Symptoms of celiac disease include diarrhea, bloating, weight loss, and anemia. These can lead to serious health complications if gluten continues to be consumed.

18.6 CELIAC TESTING

Celiac disease can be diagnosed by a blood test that looks for specific antibodies. The preferred test will look for tissue transglutaminase IgA (tTG-IgA) and total IgA. This test will be positive for 98% of people who have celiac disease and are actively consuming gluten.

A celiac patient actively produces these antibodies only if consuming gluten. For children under two years old, deamidated IgG and IgA must be included in the panel. Screening may also reflex on positive findings to other markers like Endomysial antibodies (EMA), depending on what your doctor orders.

False positive results for celiac antibodies occur infrequently in the blood tests for people with other autoimmune disorders like Hashimoto's thyroiditis, type 1 diabetes, psoriatic arthritis, rheumatoid arthritis, or autoimmune liver disease.

Celiac can be tested with a tissue biopsy during an endoscopic procedure (EGD). This continues to be the gold standard for diagnosis, because there are 2% of patients whom, even when consuming gluten actively, will test negative for tTG-IgA. For both the blood test and the biopsy, gluten must be consumed prior to the testing.

Celiac disease can also be evaluated with a genetic test for DNA markers. To have a positive result, the genetic marker test requires the presence of human leukocyte antigens (HLA-DQ2 and/or HLA-DQ8). The absence of HLA antigens can rule out the possibility of celiac disease. However, some people carry one or two of the celiac DNA strands, but not in the necessary combination to confirm a celiac diagnosis. I observe that these people are more likely to be gluten intolerant.

According to the Celiac Disease Foundation, the presence of both DQ2 and DQ8 celiac combinations are not enough to diagnose celiac. Carrying these sequences can increase the risk of celiac to 3% from the typical 1% in the general population. This test can be only used to rule out the possibility of celiac or of developing celiac disease. If you do not carry the correct gene combination, you cannot express celiac disease in your body. If you do carry the combination of DNA strands that programs celiac disease, your risk is increased but it does not confirm celiac.

Genetic testing for disease is growing quickly, and there are some very specific tests available which will confirm disease potential (for example, the testing for early onset Alzheimer's). However, genetic testing can be a grey area. There is much room for interpretation of these test results, and many tests can confirm only the *potential* for a problem. We still have a lot of data to compile before making direct correlations between a DNA sequence and a direct outcome.

Genetic testing is not invasive for the sample collection. This means that a sample can be collected with a cheek swab or saliva test, rather than a blood or biopsy test. Since your genetic material is fixed, then what you were born with is what you will always have. The result of this test does not and cannot change. You do not have to consume gluten for the HLA test. [59]

19 DIET: IDENTIFICATION OF FOOD TRIGGERS

19.1 IgG TESTING DIET

There are a few labs that offer testing for IgG foods. The functional laboratories (see index) give more specific results that correlate to patient symptoms. This is because the functional lab processes the sample differently from the standard conventional labs.

We have a disconnect with doctors who do not use functional testing. Those that run an IgG test through a conventional lab will obtain different results. Most times that I send a sample into a conventional lab for IgG foods, it comes back positive for pretty much everything. When I see this, I understand why conventional GI doctors will say that IgG testing is not helpful.

Conventional labs use a sandwich indirect immunoassay or immunocap assay as their assessment method for IgG antibodies. In my experience, this technique is too sensitive, and results in many false positive reactions. [60]

Does it even make sense that our bodies would be producing any antibody protection to foods? Our body produces IgG antibodies to protect us from infection, so in a healthy digestive system, why would we be producing quantities of antibodies against foods we are eating? I suspect that these positive IgG antibody results are a significant clue regarding gastrointestinal barrier damage. It is likely a reflection of our general underlying health and nutritional imbalances.

Functional labs use a testing method called ELISA (enzyme linked immunosorbent assay). These tests will show very clear negative and positive IgG reactions. If the entire panel is positive or moderately reactive, this indicates a generalized leaky gut response and breakdown of the gastrointestinal barrier. These test results are quantitative, which means that you can see the amount of IgG being produced for each food. The more antibodies, the stronger the adverse reaction to the food.

If the entire panel is positive, I recommend removing and challenging the main culprits: dairy, gluten, whole egg, sugar, soy, yeast and peanuts or corn. With these foods removed and the digestive system supported by supplements, the LGS can heal from the generalized reactions.

These functional panels do give some false positives and cross reaction, but they are not significant. For example, most patients show up positive for cranberry and for almond. When I order these labs, I'm looking for positives on dairy, egg, gluten, wheat, yeasts, sugar, peanut, citrus, soy, or corn. The remaining foods are indicating the degree of LGS (Leaky Gut Syndrome or breakdown in the gastrointestinal barrier). It is not necessary to eliminate them from the diet unless you have a known and clear reaction to them.

Some of the positive foods may cause symptoms that are not related to digestion. For example, someone may take dairy or gluten out of their diet and notice that their acne, eczema, psoriasis, energy level, or joint pain improves.

The World Allergy Organization has a very clear definition of IgE and non IgE reactions. I like their definitions and have included them here:

- The term "atopy" is used when individuals have an IgE sensitization as documented by IgE antibodies in serum or by a positive skin prick test.
- "Hypersensitivity" is defined as "conditions clinically resembling allergy that cause objectively reproducible symptoms or signs, initiated by exposure to a defined stimulus at a dose tolerated by normal subjects."
- "Allergy" is defined "a hypersensitivity reaction initiated by proven or strongly suspected immunologic mechanisms." [61]

Both the definitions of hypersensitivity and allergy are equivalent to what I am calling IgG (T-cell mediated) intolerance.

IgG reactions can be delayed. This means that following exposure to the food, the reaction can peak anywhere in the following 1-5 days. The delay is what makes the food panels helpful, and why I prefer to use them. If you consumed a food on Monday and have a peak reaction to it on Thursday, it's difficult to determine what food caused your symptoms. You may think it was the food you just ate, when it is a food from days ago. If you are reacting to more than one food, this complicates the problem of determining the trigger foods even more.

Because the reaction can be delayed, it takes time for the body to *stop* reacting once the food is removed. I have seen this repeatedly.

Very often I see people with extreme digestive symptoms who have been to many doctors. When I run their IgG panel, they test positive for the GI trigger foods: dairy, gluten, soy, yeast, sugar or eggs. It can take several days (or less frequently weeks) for the digestive pain to gradually calm down, but when it does, they are finally out of the debilitating pain. For additional help with this rather complex topic, I refer you back to the chapter on IgG stages of healing.

Remember, this dietary change is not for the rest of your life. Determining these IgG reactive foods is a guide to your recovery. The foods are removed, and the digestion is supported with supplements, so the healing and repair can occur. Then the foods can be added back into the diet. There may be a fixed reaction to one or two foods, or there may be a food that you either choose not to add back or that you can eat only in limited amounts. However, this should not be the rule for most foods once you've completed your GI Janel program.

My goal with each patient is to achieve a level of dietary freedom so that there is no longer a need for dietary restrictions. Most people (I'd say over 95%) who complete their GI Janel protocol can recover to this point. Some others will have a more long-term reaction to dairy or gluten and will need to limit and avoid these foods. However, the advent of greater accessibility to heirloom and ancient grain wheat may eliminate that problem and achieve the resolution of gluten intolerance. In Europe, wheat exists in the form of the ancient grain. The number of people I have seen who travel outside of North America and tolerate gluten or dairy is significant.

In my clinic, to further decrease the time required for the elimination of, food intolerances, we use a system of desensitization. We have patients coming from all over the country for food allergy desensitization. This treatment allows the immune system to recover more quickly so that the restrictive diets can be used for a shorter duration.

19.2 SKIN PATCH TESTING

Topical testing for delayed food hypersensitivities is quickly becoming my preference over IgG testing. The limitation is that it is an in-office test. The benefit is that it will pick up all the delayed cytokine reactions to a food, including the IgG pathway. The patches must remain on the skin for 3-5 days to detect food reactions.

I like this test also because it is not invasive, it's easy to use, and I can limit it to the foods that I suspect are problematic to the digestive issues. I can also expand the panel for people who have other systemic issues (rashes, acne, joint pain, fatigue), which may have a food intolerance as the underlying issue. Additionally, I can use the test to check for delayed reactions to environmental triggers.

19.3 GI FOCUSED ELIMINATION DIET

If you do not want to run the IgG test panel through a functional lab or do a skin patch test, then the simplest thing to do is eliminate the top foods that cause problems and use the soft food diet along with your GI Janel supplements.

I dislike using classic elimination diets. These are the diets where a patient eliminates all but four foods: lamb, rice, bananas and pears or uses an elemental protein powder exclusively. The diet containing these four foods is maintained for 2-4 weeks. Then foods are re-introduced one by one and reactions are recorded.

This approach is time consuming and very difficult in both the restriction and the re-introduction phases.

What I do suggest is using the soft food diet and eliminating gluten, dairy, and whole eggs (eggs as a minor ingredient in a cooked or baked food are okay). If this is not effective, then also take out sugar, yeast and soy (possibly corn and peanut).

Once symptoms have improved – and they will if you are using your supplements and eating a soft food diet (no grain carbohydrates for people who are carb reactive or intolerant) – then continue this for at least two weeks. Then begin challenging the foods one by one, a week at a time. Your body will tell you if it is ready to have this food in your diet again and at what frequency and quantity. Reserve the gluten and dairy challenge for last.

When re-introducing foods, it is imperative to do them one at a time and a week apart. For example, if you've eliminated dairy and gluten and are feeling better, don't go out and eat a pizza with cheese on it because if you react, you will not know if the gluten or the dairy is the culprit. It is also imperative to wait at least five days to monitor your reaction, which can occur immediately or within the five-day window. Doing a weekly challenge works well for tracking.

As stated previously, I consider restrictive diets like FODMAP, GAPS, SCD and SIBO to be helpful. If these are the diets you want to do, that is fine; just ensure that you are using your supplement support for repair. Additionally, ensure you have identified your personal trigger foods. If you miss the elimination of reactive or intolerant foods, you will not regain strength in your system, and ultimately the symptoms can return.

20 SOFT FOOD DIET

The soft food diet is key in the initial stages of repairing SIBO or IBS, especially if gas and bloating are a predominant part of your symptoms. Once you've removed your IgG foods, or while you're waiting on the results, it is important to take the digestive stress off your system by eating well cooked, soft foods.

Soft foods are easier to breakdown and are gentler and soothing on the digestion. This is because they are already partially broken down so they are closer to a state where they can be transported. Remember that the steps in digestion are digestion (break down), then absorption (transport from the digestive tube into the body), and elimination of waste (the leftovers).

Think of the work that your digestive system needs to do to break down a raw carrot. First, if you swallowed it without chewing well, you are sure to see pieces of carrot in your stool. What you are seeing in your stool is food that was unable to be digested by the chemical process which occurs after swallowing. Your body may be eliminating the carrot pretty close to how it was swallowed.

Now think about what it takes to digest a carrot that has been well cooked and mashed or pureed (you could add some sea salt, tamari (which is gluten free soy sauce), olive oil, butter, ghee or butter substitute for a delicious veggie dish). This carrot will be much gentler on the digestion because there is less work involved to break it down. It is also gentler because it is soft in texture rather than hard and abrasive.

In the beginning, especially for people who have a lot of gas or abdominal pain, the soft food diet is very helpful. I have even used these dietary principles to help settle symptoms for inflammatory bowel disease (IBD) like Crohn's or ulcerative colitis.

One of the problems I've encountered with patients who are struggling to find answers to their IBS or SIBO symptoms is that they try to eat a raw diet to provide more nutrients, thinking that it will help.

It is logical to think, "oh, I have a leaky gut, so I need a lot of nutrients to repair it." These people come in eating rough grains and raw foods that are making them feel worse because they are overworking an already-depleted system.

When you work with me, our goal is to repair the system so that in the long run, it will not be necessary to think about what you can or cannot eat. If you choose to eat a bowl of Brussels sprouts and raw cabbage, you can. If you want to make a veggie roll and use raw collard greens as your wrap, you can! Just don't do it until your digestion is stronger, or you'll be a gassy mess. You'll be cramping in pain as your body tries to deal with all that rough vegetable fiber.

With the soft food diet, there are fewer restrictions than the FODMAP (fermentable oligosaccharides, disaccharides, monosaccharides and polyols) and the SCD (specific carbohydrate diet). As you'll see below, if carbohydrates are tolerated when using your digestive support, I do not remove them from the diet.

How is this possible? It is because the supplements that you will be using will support digestion so that there are fewer problems with bacterial fermentation, less irritation by the foods, and less gassiness. The supplements will also work to repair the problem so that these symptoms do not return.

SIBO-specific diets are variations on the fermentable diets and will also remove easily fermentable foods. They are helpful but do the repair and support processes with them so that symptoms do not return.

20.1 THE EXPANDED SOFT FOOD DIET

When you are experiencing the symptoms of irritated digestion, it is important to remember that your gastrointestinal system is sensitive, delicate and unable to function at its normal capacity. As your system heals, we will be able to add back more variety and more whole food nutrition to your diet.

What follows is the diet I give to all patients when we first start to work together. With these dietary changes, and your prescribed supplements, you will experience some immediate relief from the acute and painful events that occur.

Once we have identified any possible food intolerance/infections, this diet will be modified to accommodate for them.

If you are not doing IgG blood testing or the skin patch test, then eliminate the following:

- Cow dairy (DF)
- Gluten (GF) – wheat, spelt, kamut, barley, rye, triticale
- Whole eggs and mayonnaise (egg as a minor ingredient is ok)
- Sugar
- Legumes (beans, hummus)
- Soybeans – tamari soy sauce is okay
- Possibly corn and peanut

Guidelines:

- Avoid whole grains
- Avoid crunchy foods / nuts
- Avoid raw foods
- Avoid fried and fermented foods (kombucha/tempeh)
- Avoid strong spices
- Avoid tomato, garlic, onion, peppers, broccoli, cauliflower, cabbage, Brussels sprouts
- Stop any probiotics unless your doctor has checked them.
- Use Your prescribed supplement with all meals and snacks as directed
- Limit or avoid alcohol, coffee, and carbonated beverages and strong tea.
- Use date sugar, stevia, honey, maple syrup, or coconut sugar in small amounts.
- Avoid large or heavy meals. Eat meals slowly & chew very well.
- Rest after eating if possible.

Choose from the following for your meals and snacks:

- Carbohydrates, in the form of white potato, yam, sweet potato, carrots, beets, squash or, pumpkin. Any well-cooked version of this, but mashed or pureed is ideal, or try baked home fries.

- Home fries: Cut russet potatoes or any root veggie into wedges or fries and put in a bowl. Coat well with olive or avocado oil and salt. Mix well. Bake on a cookie sheet at 425 degrees for 20 minutes, then flip them over and bake for another 20-40 minutes to a golden brown
- Cooked soft, leafy greens (spinach or chard)
- Oats, oatmeal, rice cereal, quinoa cereal
- Soft gluten-free cereal, pancakes, breads
- White rice, rice cakes
- Quinoa, teff or rice products
- Polenta, gluten-free corn bread
- Rice or quinoa noodles
- Corn tortillas
- Baked or stewed: apples, strawberries, pears
- Apple sauce, pear sauce
- Ripe mango, papaya, banana, berries, melon, peach
- Ripe avocado
- Guacamole

If you experience more bloating/gas/pain with grains, then stick to the non- grain items in the above list.

Protein sources:
- Organic animal protein. Choose bland meats like turkey, chicken, fish, beef, buffalo, or lamb.
- Cheese/dairy product made from goat milk, sheep milk, buffalo milk, hemp, coconut, rice, or nuts
- Protein powders: rice, bone broth, chia or hemp hearts
- Nut butters: cashew, hazelnut, almond, sesame, pecan, or macadamia

For flavor, use fresh-pressed oils like avocado oil, olive oil, sesame oil, dairy, gluten and egg free earth balance, spreads and dressings, ghee, nut butter, seed butters, tamari (gluten free soy sauce), sea salt, mild herbs and spices (rosemary, thyme, oregano, basil, and cinnamon).

Easy soup: Boil your vegetables until soft. Blend until smooth in blender and add 1 tsp. of "better than bullion" or other bullion. Mix to a smooth soup and add canned coconut milk or grass-fed butter or earth balance spread.

Snacks:

- Rice cakes with fruit or spreads
- Plantain chips (chew well)
- Dairy-free pudding and yogurts
- Fruit sauces
- Fruit and nut butters or dairy free spreads

20.2 SUMMARY OF THE SOFT FOOD DIET

The main features of the soft-food diet are:

- No raw foods
- No crunchy foods (soft only)
- No high-fiber foods
- Eliminate the following: gluten, animal dairy, whole eggs, soy, commercial yeast, sugar and possibly corn and peanut, unless IgG-negative or until symptoms calm and you can challenge them for their impact.

20.3 LEVELS OF SOFT FOOD DIET

20.3.1 Level One: Constant Symptoms

This is a classic SIFO or yeast-overgrowth symptom that is often coupled with SIBO (bacterial overgrowth). Some people get bloating and gassy symptoms even without food. Some people get symptoms just by drinking plain water. I certainly had that experience twenty years ago when embarking on my own journey with IBS/SIBO/SIFO. In fact, I remember that even when I ate *nothing*, I would start to bloat up like clockwork around noon every day. I experienced painful bloating, distention and borborygmus (noisy intestinal gas), which is a signature symptom of both SIBO and SIFO coupled with overgrowth in the large intestine. It is also indicative of pancreatic deficiency and the inability to summon the digestive capacity beyond the first meal of the day.

If this describes you, I'm so sorry that this is where you are. It's scary, and I understand it because I was there too.

Not to worry! Follow this simple diet below, add in GI Janel support, and your symptoms can begin to dissipate. This diet will be very simple at first. I have been reading some online accounts of symptoms and frustration with diets. Those that impact me the most are the people who have been struggling with restrictive diets for years only to find that their symptoms remain the same regardless of the diet they try.

GI Janel One will get to the cause of your problems, and once you reach the higher doses, your diet can expand to healthier, whole foods.

Bone Broths

Use 2 pounds or more of healthy bones. This means bones from animals that were raised without antibiotics and hormones. It's even better if they are from animals given organic feed, or are grass fed or free range.

The healthier the life of the animal, the richer in nutrients they are for you to eat. Buy from a local butcher or farmer's market that features grass fed, organic animals. You can even buy premade and packaged bone broth online.

If you cannot get organic bones, then just get whatever you can from a regular store. Right now, it's simply important to have something that you can eat without symptoms.

This diet is different than the low-fermentable diets. I advocate the addition of sweeteners and carbohydrates right in the beginning. This is because you will be taking your GI Janel Digest

Formula and your GI Janel One right from the beginning. These will increase your ability to eat the foods below without symptoms.

Recipe for Bone Broth

- Roast your bones in the oven for 30 minutes at 350° F to increase their flavor

- Place the bones in a 5-gallon stock pot. Pour filtered water over the bones to cover them.

- Add 2 tsp sea salt

- Bring to a boil and then simmer until done. This will take several hours. As the broth cooks, remove and discard any foam that floats to the top. The more organic your bones are, the less of this there will be. Taste and add more salt as needed.

- Remove from the heat, cool, then strain.

- The broth will keep for five days if refrigerated, or you can freeze it.

- As you gain confidence eating bone broth, you can start to add meats (beef, chicken, turkey, lamb, bison or white fish to your broth)

Grains

There may be one type of grain that you will tolerate. For most people, this is white rice. If well-cooked white rice still causes symptoms, try quinoa. If well-cooked quinoa causes symptoms, I would advise taking grains out altogether (this would be a paleo diet minus whole eggs and with the addition of starchy veggies.) Do not worry that rice is not SIBO legal. Please, just try it. If you're carb-intolerant, you'll know soon enough. But 90% of you will be able to tolerate rice and this will open your world of limited diet choices.

To cook rice or quinoa

- Rinse the grain well with cold water until the water is clear.
- Drain.
- Add water in ratio of 1 to 1.5 (e.g. 1 cup of grain to 1.5 cups of water, or 2 cups of grain to 3 cups of water).
- Bring to a boil, stir and cover with a lid.
- Reduce heat and simmer on the lowest heat for 20 min.
- After 20 min, turn off the heat, leaving the lid on, and let stand for 20 more min.
- Once cooked, mix with bouillon or gluten free soy, alternate butter or nut butter for a savory meal. Mix with fruit puree or cacao and sweetener for a sweet dish.

Congee

Congee is a staple in the Chinese diet. It is basically a rice soup. If you have tried white rice and it seems to be calming rather than irritating to your system, this will be a good option for you.

- Wash 2 cups of white rice until water runs clear.
- Add 6-8 cups of water.
- Add 2 tsp of sea salt to taste.
- Bring to a boil and then reduce heat and simmer for 2 or more hours until rice is very soft and is like a thick soup. Add more water if needed.
- Add more salt to taste or add tamari (gluten-free soy sauce) or earth balance original spread.

Rice Pudding

If you tolerate rice well, then rice pudding is another soothing option.

- 1 cup of white rice rinsed until water runs clear.
- Add 4 cups of almond, coconut, nut, rice milk or other alternative milk (non-cow dairy) or cow dairy if tolerated.

Bring to a boil, then simmer over low heat to make a thick pudding, adding more milk as needed. When you get braver, you can try adding honey, maple syrup, stevia and maybe some cooked fruits.

Root Veggies

White potato, yams, sweet potato, potato, parsnip, turnip, beet, carrot

- Eat well cooked, mashed and pureed root veggies. You may be able to tolerate these lightly fried or baked in oil.
- Home fries: Cut russet potatoes or any root veggie into wedges or fries and put in a bowl. Coat well with olive or avocado oil and salt. Mix well. Bake on a cookie sheet at 425 degrees for 20 minutes, then flip them over and bake for another 20-40 minutes to a golden brown.

Soft Veggies

Spinach, swish chard

- Steam until very soft and eat these at first in small amounts

For any of the dishes, you can add flavor with tamari, sea salt, nut butters, avocado, Bragg Liquid Amino, ghee, grass fed butter or dairy free spread (we like earth balance original)

Soft Fruit

One serving a day maximum to start. Do not eat if the fruit sugars cause digestive symptoms.

Ripe, mashed banana, berries, mango, papaya, avocado

Hard Fruit

Apples and pears

- Bake or Steam then puree or mash adding in sea salt, ghee or dairy free spread or sweeteners (honey, maple syrup, coconut sugar, stevia, agave)

Avoid

If you don't want to do the IgG food panel or patch test, you are best to avoid:

- Dairy
- Gluten
- Whole eggs (eggs as a minor ingredient are okay)
- Soy
- Sugar
- Yeast (yeast is added to a lot of packaged foods and is in bread and beer. The more commercial a packaged product is, the nastier the yeast)
- Peanut (for some people)
- Corn (for some people)

20.3.2   Level Two: Symptoms come and go

If you do not have symptoms constantly or with every meal, you'll have more flexibility with what you eat. On the second level of the soft food diet, continue with the ideas in the first level while adding the modifications below. Chew your food 20 times before swallowing.

A soft food diet is not the time to be attempting to extract nutrition from raw or whole foods. This is the time to eat processed, non-fibrous foods with low residue that will not annoy your system. Don't worry; once you're feeling better from the diet and supplements, you will again be able to expand your diet choices to raw, whole foods, and even gluten and dairy for some.

Soups

Start with the bone broth recipe above but add in organic meats (lamb, beef, turkey, chicken, bison, white fish) and well-cooked root veggies. Try some mild spices like oregano, basil, rosemary. If you don't have time to make bone broth, start with a basic chicken bouillon or other stock, and add your meats and root veggies and gluten free grains if tolerated.

Stock can be purchased in stores in cubes, powders or pastes that only require the addition of water to make your stock. They tend to be quite salty, but this is not going to be a problem unless you have blood pressure issues directly related to salt intake. If this is the case, purchase low sodium brands.

It is best to make your own soups rather than buying pre-made or canned. The preservatives, gums and thickeners added to commercial products may irritate your digestion.

Rice, Corn or Quinoa

As stated, do not eat these grains if they are not tolerated. If they are (and they will be for 90% of people) you can start to experiment with soft corn tortillas, soft crackers and breads made from these gluten free grains. You may also experiment with ancient or heirloom wheat products but choose the white-flour types rather than the whole wheat until your digestion is stronger. For example: heirloom (ancient) wheat or spelt French or Sourdough breads instead of multigrain.

Meats

Any of the meats listed above: beef, chicken, turkey, bison, lamb, and white fish

Nut butters

Experiment with small servings like by the teaspoon amounts of butter made from nuts (cashew, sesame, pistachios, hazelnuts, almonds, walnuts, pine nuts)

If this goes well, you can make your own butters simply by grinding up nuts in a food processer and adding nut oils and salts if needed.

Nut Milks

You can make nut milks, which are delicious and can be frozen for a treat

- ¼ cup nuts
- 1 cup of filtered water

Blend together until smooth and use in your rice pudding or cereal or as a drink. This milk can also be frozen. Add fruit for flavor or sweeteners: honey, stevia, coconut sugar, maple syrup, or cacao for an easy dessert or snack.

If your symptoms are better with this level of the soft food diet and supplement protocol, then you can go back to the expanded version of the soft food diet.

20.4 CARB INTOLERANCE

Doing a carbohydrate challenge is helpful to distinguish carbohydrate intolerance from other carbohydrate issues like gluten intolerance. It is quite simple to do, and your body will tell you what it likes. Thankfully, like everything we've been looking at when considering IBS and SIBO, carbohydrate intolerance and gluten intolerance have the potential to be resolved over time. (Celiac disease does not.)

Carbohydrates are prevalent in many foods. It's easy to remember that in general, carbohydrates grow in the ground and proteins walk around.

Carbohydrates include grains, vegetables, fruits, nuts and legumes. The most concentrated carbohydrates are the grain-based carbohydrates, processed foods and sugars. This includes gluten grains: wheat, spelt, rye, barley, kamut, farro, durum, bulgur and semolina.

It also includes gluten-free grains: rice, quinoa, amaranth, buckwheat, oats and teff. Carbohydrate intolerance occurs due to a deficiency in the enzymes that break down carbohydrates. Carbohydrates (starches) are broken down initially by the enzymes that your pancreas releases into the first part of the small intestine. Then they travel through the small intestine as the enzymes work on them, breaking them down more and more until they reach the middle to end of the small intestine, where they are transported across the gastrointestinal barrier into the body. At this stage, the grain starches are broken down into their smallest pre-digested form, disaccharides of maltose, which is a double glucose chain.

The final breakdown of a carbohydrate is accomplished by enzymes produced in the brush border in the small intestine. The only units that can be transported across the cells of a healthy intestine are monosaccharides, which are the smallest building blocks of carbohydrates. ("Mono" means one and "di" means two.)

There are only three monosaccharides that build carbohydrates: glucose, galactose and fructose. Glucose and galactose are transported across the gastrointestinal barrier by a mechanism that is sodium-dependent, and fructose is transported by simple diffusion.

At the brush border of the small intestine (gastrointestinal barrier), disaccharidase enzymes break the disaccharides into monosaccharides, which are then small enough to be transported through the intestinal cell and into your body. These enzymes are the last step in carbohydrate digestion.

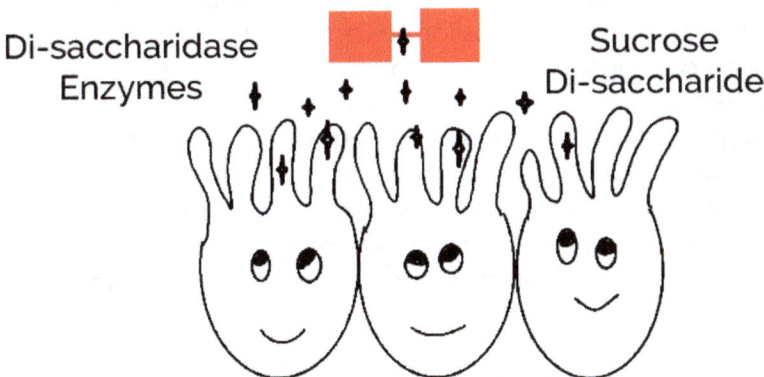

Figure 20.1 Disaccharide split into monosaccharide

- The enzyme *maltase* splits maltose into two molecules of glucose.
- The enzyme *lactase* splits lactose into glucose and galactose.
- The enzyme *sucrase* splits sucrose into glucose and fructose.

But if there is a deficiency of disaccharide enzymes (or pancreatic enzymes), then you will have disaccharide or larger carbohydrate chains loitering in the small intestine that cannot be transported across and into your body. Since this is a sugar in a dark, warm place with bacteria and yeasts, guess what happens? The little microbes gobble up the disaccharides and produce *fermentation and gas*! Doesn't that sound like your SIBO and IBS symptom? Even with normal populations of bacteria and yeasts, gas and bloating can occur with an enzyme deficiency and gastrointestinal barrier damage. It is compounded, however, when SIBO (small intestinal bacterial overgrowth) or SIFO (small intestinal yeast overgrowth) are present.

Now, why would you have a deficiency of disaccharide splitting enzymes?

For the same reason that you would have a deficiency of probiotics or an overgrowth of unwanted bacteria or yeast. For the same reason that you developed food intolerances. The system is not healthy, it is not strong and cannot accomplish selective absorption. Digestion is weakened. The gastrointestinal barrier is damaged and permeable. The immune system is sensitized and reactive. With a damaged gastrointestinal barrier, the digestive system is subject to constant inflammation and exposure to food triggers. It's a vicious cycle. It is imperative that the gastrointestinal barrier separates the gut contents from the immune system. It is imperative that the gastrointestinal barrier acts as a selective membrane for fully digested food transport into the body.

The immune system cannot interface with the intestinal contents without becoming sensitized to foods and creating an ongoing inflammatory process when these foods are eaten again.

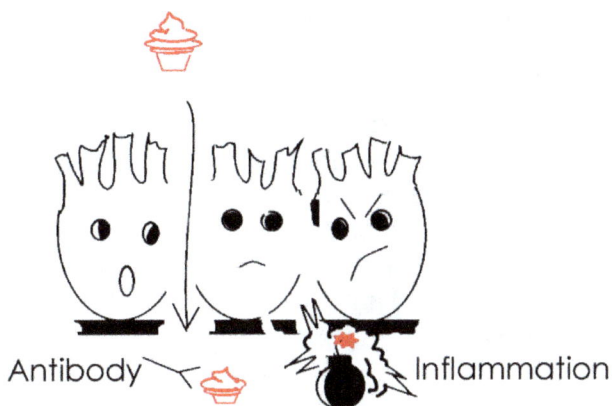

Figure 20.2
Gastrointestinal barrier and antibody formation

Antibody

Inflammation

For patients with SIBO or SIFO, monosaccharides will also be a problem. Since these simple sugars, glucose, fructose, and galactose, can be absorbed directly without further breakdown, then there should be no carb intolerance with them. However, overgrowth of bacteria and yeast can still ferment these and create gas. A damaged gastrointestinal barrier can also be unable to efficiently transport monosaccharides. If monosaccharides cause symptoms, it's likely that damage to the gastrointestinal barrier in addition to bacterial (SIBO) or yeast (SIFO) overgrowth is your diagnosis.

Testing for monosaccharide intolerance (due to GI damage or bacterial or yeast overgrowth) is possible for you to do at home.

Eat some honey, pure fructose or pure glucose (also called dextrose). Do this when your symptoms are calm, and see if you get any gas, bloating, abdominal pain, diarrhea or constipation. If you do, then chances are your primary problem is SIBO or SIFO.

To summarize: You can have SIBO and SIFO symptoms without bacteria or yeast overgrowth when the gastrointestinal barrier is damaged.

You can have SIBO and SIFO symptoms without bacterial or yeast overgrowth when you have food intolerances and gastrointestinal barrier damage.

You can have SIBO and SIFO symptoms without bacterial or yeast overgrowth when there is a compromise in the secretion of acid from the stomach cells, pancreatic enzymes from the pancreas and bile from the gallbladder.

You can have a SIBO and SIFO diagnosis and positive breath test for SIBO and have concomitant gastrointestinal barrier damage. In this case, once you complete your antibiotic and antifungal treatment, the symptoms persist or return. The chances of having SIBO without gastrointestinal barrier damage or digestive deficiency are highly unlikely. It is the GI function weakness that allows for the overgrowth.

20.5 FRUCTOSE INTOLERANCE (MALABSORPTION)

Hereditary fructose Intolerance is a lifelong, serious condition caused by an enzyme deficiency. It is a problem with fructose metabolism following transport into the body and is diagnosed in infancy. It is life threatening and if not diagnosed will lead to death.

Acquired fructose intolerance, which is synonymous with malabsorption, has its origins in gastrointestinal barrier compromise or overgrowth.

Now that we understand carb breakdown and transport, and gastrointestinal barriers and fermentation, we can talk about acquired fructose intolerance. Remember that fructose is a monosaccharide and is ready for absorption without further breakdown. Common symptoms of intolerance include gassiness, bloating, diarrhea and fatigue.

Doesn't this sound like IBS/SIBO?

The gas and the bloating are fermentation symptoms as the fructose sits in the intestine. The diarrhea is an osmotic irritation. The osmotic diarrhea is the same thing that happens when you eat too much alcohol sugar like xylitol. Have you ever read the package of a low-carb candy sweetened with xylitol or erythritol? Too much will give you diarrhea.

Fructose is transported by facilitated diffusion and does not require ion transfer like the other two monosaccharides. Acquired fructose intolerance results primarily from damage to the gastrointestinal barrier or SIBO/SIFO. All these problems should be repaired and improved following the GI Janel program. I have outlined how to deal with IBS and SIBO in the treatment chapters of this book. [62]

20.6 HISTAMINE, SALICYLATE AND NON-FERMENTABLE DIETS

I do my best to avoid these diets in my practice, unless a patient really wants to try them. However, I find them very restrictive, as they eliminate many healthy foods.

I prefer to determine the specific irritants, heal the system, treat hypersensitivities with desensitization, and then re-introduce a whole-food, healthy diet as soon as possible.

20.7 CARB CHALLENGE

Once you're on the soft food diet, have eliminated trigger foods, and are taking your supportive GI Janel supplements, your system will be calm enough to do a carbohydrate challenge.

It makes the most sense to challenge a gluten-free carbohydrate, so you'll know if you are reacting to the gluten or to the carbohydrate.

When your symptoms are calm, eat ½ cup of well cooked, white rice (basmati or jasmine are best).

In general, if the challenge does not cause any symptoms, then you can add soft, gluten-free carbohydrates to your diet as instructed in the soft food diet information. Rice is very soothing and healing to digestion and it helps to support the mucous layer of the intestine. Rice is also a gentle bulking fiber which will help your stools to move. If rice causes constipation, ensure you are drinking electrolyte water (Recharge or Nuun hydration tablets) throughout your day. In terms of gluten free products, the less processed they are, the more easily they can be digested. Some gluten-free breads contain gums and thickeners that cause symptoms that will mimic IBS/SIBO symptoms.

21 IBS/SIBO Affect the Immune and Endocrine System

Quite simply, if your digestive system is chronically inflamed (expressed by the symptoms of abdominal pain, gas, bloating, diarrhea or constipation) then your immune system is over-active in the digestive process. This occurs mainly because of food intolerances or hidden infections that your immune system is fighting (like yeast and bacteria that are not necessarily pathogenic but are irritating). If your immune system is occupied trying to protect you from foods or hidden infections, then there are less available resources to fight off infections like colds or flu viruses.

Long term IBS/SIBO symptoms can take a toll on the endocrine system, mainly on the adrenal glands, which are responsible for mitigating stresses in our bodies. Chronic digestive stress means chronic adrenal response which in time can make this system weak or compromised. The serious medical term for adrenal compromise is Addison's disease. This disease state renders the adrenals either nonfunctional or only partially operational. Addison's is serious: it requires pharmaceutical intervention and it is life threatening.

Adrenal weakness, on the other hand, results in symptoms such as fatigue, anxiety, insomnia, and reproductive hormone imbalance. It is disruptive and can be associated with fibromyalgia or chronic fatigue. By resolving the ongoing symptoms of IBS/SIBO, a major stressor is removed from the body. Typically, once the digestive symptoms are resolved, supporting the adrenal glands with nutrients, supplements and lifestyle measures will be helpful to improve secondary conditions caused by the ongoing digestive stress.

22 GI Janel Treatment

The treatment consists of three components, all of which are needed to eliminate symptoms and repair your system for permanent resolution.

Diet

Level one soft food diet

Level two soft food diet

Expanded soft food diet

Digestive Support Supplements

GI Janel Digest A or

GI Janel Digest B or

GI Janel Digest C

Cell Repair and Overgrowth Elimination Supplements:

GI Jan-Aloe

GI Janel One

Constipation support if needed

GI Janel AM / BM

23 GI JANEL ONE, THE SCIENCE

23.1 GI JANEL ONE- A BRIEF OVERVIEW

GI Janel One is formulated to treat the three key aspects that are required to relieve gas and bloating in IBS and SIBO: microbiome balance, microbiome distribution and cellular repair.

The microbiome balance and distribution are important so that unwanted bacteria or yeast no longer ferment your foods causing gassy bloating.

Cellular repair is important so that the cells can effectively release the proper enzymes to digest and selectively absorb the building blocks of food. Cellular repair is also important to re-establish the gastrointestinal barrier. A strong gastrointestinal barrier will keep your immune system separate from the food contents digesting in the intestine. The immune system and digestive content should never interface. They require the intact gastrointestinal barrier to keep them separate. Inappropriate interfaces between the digestive contents and the immune system lead to food intolerances and a chronic inflammatory response. Repair and temporary avoidance will achieve symptom relief so that you are no longer intolerant to many foods.

GI Janel One is the most powerful and successful treatment that I have used in the past 20 years for the resolution of SIBO/IBS and SIFO.

It is gentle and effective as a natural antifungal and bacteriostatic agent, and it is essential for tissue strength and repair. GI Janel One contains the third most-common mineral in your body composition, sulfur. Sulfur is not stored in the body and so you must have a constant intake to maintain healthy levels of sulfur for tissue repair. GI Janel One requires a gradual dose titration (slow increase) to resolve gas and bloating. Because of the microbiome acclimation in the initial stages, you may pass more gas. This is normal and will decline.

GI Janel One is well-tolerated for people with sulfite intolerance. GI Janel One soothes and heals the mucous layer of the intestine with gentle, demulcent herbs. It also contains a water-soluble fiber called acacia, which promotes regular, formed bowels for cases of either diarrhea or constipation.

GI Janel One is not to be use in cases of hypersensitivity or allergy. As with all treatments, consult your health care provider prior to taking in pregnancy.

23.2 DIGESTIVE REPAIR

GI Janel One contains sulfur in the form of MSM (methylsulfonylmethane). MSM is a compound of sulfur that is biologically available to our bodies. MSM is made of two methyl groups (CH3) and two oxygens (O) bound to a sulfur (S).

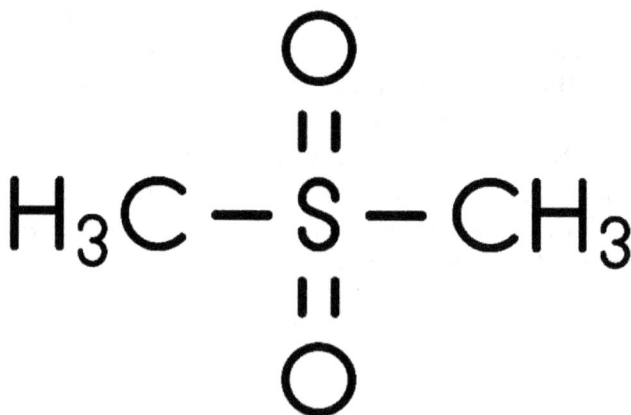

$$H_3C - \overset{\displaystyle \overset{O}{\|}}{\underset{\displaystyle \underset{O}{\|}}{S}} - CH_3$$

Figure 23.1
Chemical structure of MSM

MSM provides the sulfur required for the building of glycosaminoglycans (GAG). GAGs are the basis of connective tissue, and connective tissue forms the gastrointestinal barrier. GAGs are responsible for the structure of every connective tissue in the body, from microscopic membranes all the way to the bones and cartilage.

The main GAGs are heparin sulfate, chondroitin sulfate, keratin sulfate and dermatan sulfate. These GAGs are combined to form collagen.

There are many subcategories of connective tissue, but when considering the GI tract, the connective tissues structures include dense irregular and loose connective tissue, desmosomes, and actin filaments. GAGs form the collagen, and the collagen forms the connective tissue. [63] [64]

All glycosaminoglycans (GAG) contain sulfur except for hyaluronic acid. Chondroitin sulfate primarily forms the basement membrane of the intestine. The basement membrane is the outer coating around the tube. This basement membrane along with the cell-to-cell connections are important structures of the gastrointestinal barrier. Remember that the gastrointestinal barrier is imperative for the separation of the digestive contents from the immune system. If the immune system can interact with the digestive contents through a damaged gastrointestinal barrier, it will want to protect you from what it will read as foreign proteins digesting in the intestine. This is the beginning of an inflammatory process. [65]

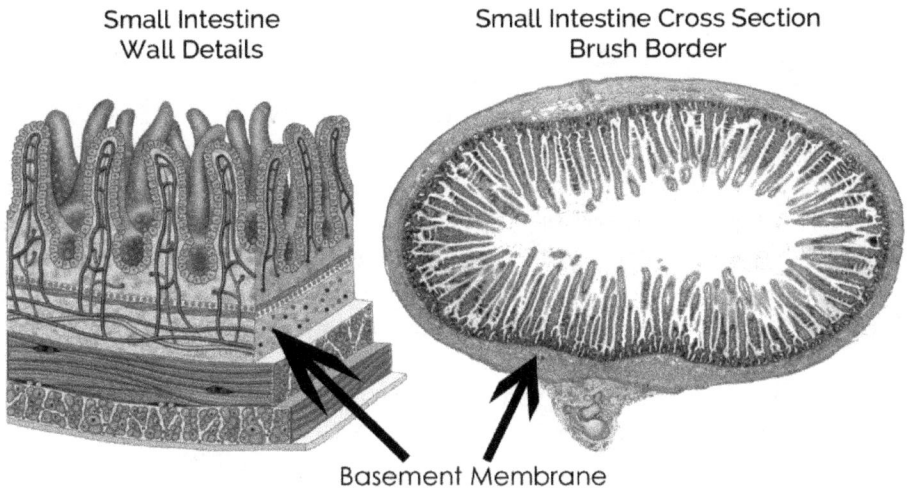

Small Intestine
Wall Details

Small Intestine Cross Section
Brush Border

Basement Membrane

Figure 23.2 *Cross Section of Small Intestine with an Intact Basement Membrane*

The three-dimensional structure of collagen relies on disulfide bonds. Disulfide bonds are made of sulfur that connects two amino acids. The amino acids that form these bonds are two cysteines linked through their sulfur to form cystine. You can picture it like two sulfurs holding hands.

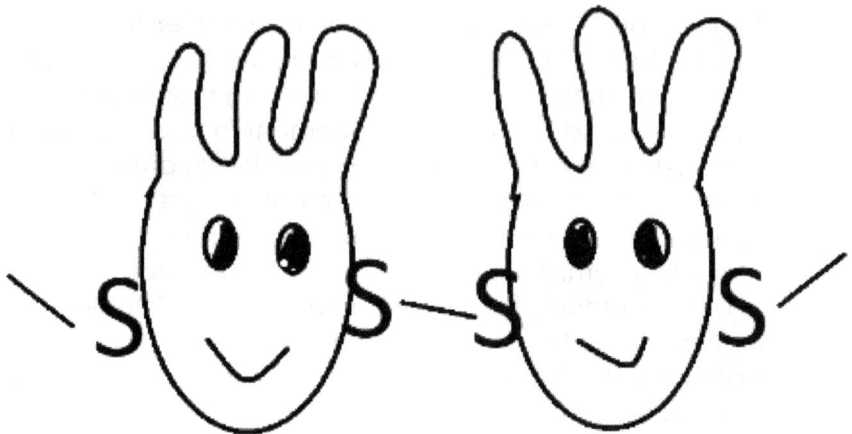

Figure 23.3 The Disulfide Bond

There are only three main bonds that give three-dimensional structure to proteins in the body, and disulfide bonds are one of them. The others are salt bridges and hydrogen bonds. The more disulfide bonds there are, the harder the structure. For example, fingernails have very high levels of disulfide bonds. Skin and intestinal lining have fewer bonds, allowing them to stretch and move then return to their original positions. This flexible collagen is used to build the digestive system, including the valves that separate the stomach from the small intestine and the small from the large intestine. [66]

The strength of our hair is due to disulfide bonds. The content of sulfur in hair is extremely high to provide the large number of disulfide bonds required to give hair its great tensile strength. These disulfide bonds are so strong that virtually intact hair has been recovered from ancient Egyptian tombs.[67]

The junctions between the intestinal cells rely on sulfur. In the digestive tract, these are called occluding junctions. Actin and keratin filaments primarily secure the junctions on the inside of the cell (in the cytoplasm) and between the cells, the junctions are maintained by cadherin filaments.[68]

Actin and keratin are formed from the sulfur-rich proteins containing the amino acid cysteine (or cystine, which is two cysteine amino acids linked by a disulfide bond) and methionine. Actin filaments promote motility, making sulfur an important element for cell membrane permeability and elasticity.[69]

There are polyamines (small proteins) called spermidine, putrescine and spermine, which are involved in the healing of blunted or damaged small intestinal cells. The synthesis of these small proteins from putrescine and arginine is sulfur dependent. When experimental models are given these proteins, the healing of the small intestinal cells is accelerated. These molecules appear to be growth factors, necessary for cellular division (repair).[70]

Sulfur can transport oxygen into cells. This is also an important aspect of cellular repair, as this intracellular oxygen is essential to healthy cellular regeneration.

To summarize, GI Janel One contains sulfur in the form of MSM as an essential building block for the repair of cell-to-cell connections and the cellular basement membranes. The sulfur can also be used to produce the protective mucous lining, improve motility, cell permeability and elasticity in the digestive system. [71]

Other helpful GI repair products include concentrated aloe mucopolysaccharides, Deglycyrrhizinated licorice (DGL), marshmallow root (althea), Sacromyces boulardii, slippery elm (Ulmus), zinc, vitamin A, essential fatty acids, and B vitamins.

I rarely prescribe the follow treatments, which are commonly used in functional GI medicine: okra, N-acetyl glucosamine, mastic gum, mucin, glutamine, guar gum and immunoglobulins, as I have seen them irritate and cause cramping or diarrhea if used before the system is strong enough.

23.3 Microbiome Balance

GI Janel One can gently and naturally reduce yeast and unwanted bacteria in the intestine. Historically, sulfur was one of the first antifungal medications. Sulfur is the main antifungal used in organic farming.[72] Sulfur is used as a natural antimicrobial in the food industry.

I have seen the bacteriostatic nature of MSM sulfur, at a high dose, decrease and eliminate the overgrowth of bacteria and yeast in the small intestines. This eliminates SIBO and SIFO symptoms.

MSM is known to possess antimicrobial effects against organisms such as giardia lamblia, trichomonas vaginalis, and fungi (yeast). The suggested mechanism is that MSM binds to surface receptor sites, blocking the interaction of infectious species and host.[73]

The intestines are an anaerobic environment (there is no oxygen). In an anaerobic environment, sulfate reducing bacteria (SRB), use elemental sulfur or sulfate as the receptor in the electron transport chain that ultimately provides them with energy.

Intestinal microbes can ferment the products of carbohydrate breakdown (SIBO), called pyruvate. Sulfate and sulfur are the electron receptors in the final step of this process. The result is the production of energy along with ethanol and gases. I theorize that the reason for the increased gassiness in the beginning of the GI Janel One treatment is an acclimation of the unwanted species to the presence of therapeutic levels of sulfur. Eventually when the sulfur levels reach a bacteriostatic level, they will be effective in the goal of microbiome balance. This is the reason for the gradual increase of GI Janel One. This is also the reason that the gassiness dissipates over time with the gradual increasing levels of GI Janel One. You are removing the unwanted bacteria and can have less gas produced. [74]

Providing adequate levels of sulfur to the body can stop the compensation mechanism in the gut that is promoting the sulfur-reducing bacteria (SRB). When the body has the sulfur it needs, there is no longer a requirement for the additional sulfur gas-producing bacteria to overgrow. So, these SRB die off and the microbiome distribution of both the large and small intestine benefit. The overgrowth of methane and hydrogen gas-producing species are then reduced because of this shift. I've seen this work many times in practice. I'll test a patient who is positive for SIBO. We'll treat with therapeutic doses of GI Janel One, then repeat the breath test once symptoms resolve, and the SIBO is eradicated. My current working theory is that the microbiome balance is a result of replenishing the fundamental sulfur needs of the body.

The sulfate-reducing bacteria are Desulfovibrio, Desulfobacter, Desulfomonas, Desulfobulbus, and Desulfotomaculum. Other species that create hydrogen sulfide are streptococcus, fusobacterium, salmonella, Enterobacter, and helicobacter.[75]

Both the methanogens that produce methane gases and the SRB can complete for the available hydrogen made by the hydrogen dominant SIBO species. It's a complex ecosystem. Not all these gases are bad – the imbalance of them causing gassy symptoms is what is bad. In fact, hydrogen sulfide can regulate motility and inflammation. It can contribute to short-chain fatty acid production and decrease damage from NSAID use. Unlike the carbohydrate-loving methanogens, SRB can use fats as their fuel source.

Some classic hydrogen sulfide overgrowth symptoms include body pain and rashes, belching, hot gasses, and a rotten egg smell in the flatulence. When the SRB overgrow in the small intestine, diarrhea is more of an issue. When the SRB overgrow in the large intestine, constipation becomes more dominant.

There will soon be a breath test available to detect the overgrowth of sulfur-reducing bacteria in the intestine.

GI Janel One is bacteriostatic (it inhibits bacterial growth). This differs from sulfur in the antibiotic form, which is bactericidal (it *kills* bacteria). MSM and the antibiotic form of sulfa are not the same. You can read about this in the chapter on forms of sulfur. You cannot have a sulfur intolerance or allergy. This is impossible as sulfur is essential to life.

The bacteriostatic sulfur content of GI Janel One is essential to its function. It can help the body inhibit the overgrowth of unwanted species without sacrificing the desired microbiome. This microbiome shift occurs simultaneously with the increased system strength provided by GI Janel One. The result is a balance of microbiota required for healthy digestion and symptom resolution.[76]

Sulfur has long been known as an antifungal and therefore I use it to combat overgrowth of yeasts in the small (SIFO) and large intestine (colon). Some plants can even produce their own sulfur to protect them from fungal growth.[77]

If we can stop the growth and proliferation of the unwanted species and provide the intestine with what it needs to heal, then the immune system can regain its strength enough to take care of the rest. This requires more research, but it is certainly what I have seen repeatedly in clinical practice. I have witnessed patients with chronic gas and bloating pain who, after ramping up and maintaining their GI Janel One dose, experience complete and permanent resolution of these symptoms. I have been following some of these people for over a decade, and their symptoms remain resolved.

23.4 OTHER FUNCTIONS OF SULFUR IN THE BODY

The body uses sulfur for repair and for detoxification. The sulfur amino acids cysteine and cystine are essential components for building and repairing your tissues and protein structure. Sulfur supports enzyme reactions in the body and protein synthesis.

Sulfur is needed to make collagen which is the building block of the connective tissue that keeps your skin, hair, nails and joints youthful, healthy and strong. Keratin contains sulfur, and this gives strength, rigidity and shape to skin, hair and nails. In fact, breaking and remaking of the disulfide bonds is how a hair perm is able to create curls. The disulfide bonds of the straight hair are broken and re-formed after the hair is wrapped around curlers. This permanently curls the hair.

Fur and feathers also contain sulfur for strength. The high sulfur content of eggs is present for feather development in birds.[78]

Mucopoly-saccharides which give support to connective tissue can contain sulfur.

The four sulfur-containing amino acids (cysteine, methionine, homocysteine and taurine) are necessary for many enzyme reactions, and are involved in protein synthesis (repair), oxygen utilization, free radical quenching (antioxidant) and liver detoxification (using L-cysteine and glutathione).

Sulfur is essential for the formation of collagen and disulfide bonds throughout the body. Sulfur is the basis for strong, cellular connections between the intestinal cells that form the important gastrointestinal barrier. Sulfur is integral to the basement membrane on which the cells of the intestine sit, and that separates the tube of digestion from the immune system. In this way, GI Janel One provides elements that are essential for the repair of the selective membrane nature of the intestine.

Collagen is also necessary for the repair of the sphincter, which separates the small from the large intestine (this can be damaged and back flowing in SIBO).

The Weston Price Foundation, one of the primary research bodies for nutrition, has an enormous amount of information on sulfur and the effects of sulfur-deficient diets. According to the foundation, sulfur deficiency due to soil depletion and processed food diets is associated with obesity, glucose metabolism issues, metabolic syndrome and atherosclerosis. They also suggest that adequate levels of sulfur may be helpful in preventing or delaying the onset of dementia. There is very detailed, analytical information available on the Weston Price website.[79]

To summarize the importance of sulfur:

- It is a structural element for all connective tissue
- It creates the tertiary (three dimensional) structure of the body
- It is required for detoxification in the form of glutathione

- It is required for taurine synthesis which is essential for our cardiovascular system, muscles, and our central nervous system.
- It binds together insulin amino acid chains.[80]

23.5 GENETIC MUTATIONS AND SULFUR USE

If you are having any trouble taking sulfur in the form of MSM, it is good idea to check for CBS or cystathione beta synthase mutations. This enzyme aids in the conversion of homocysteine to cystathione. If the enzyme is not working properly due to a genetic mutation, then it has the potential to kick off excess ammonia and hydrogen sulfide or increase sulfites in the body. People with these mutations may need lower doses for longer terms to get the repair benefits of GI Janel One. I address this also in the dosing chapter for GI Janel One and in the section on sulfur intolerance.

Problems with conversion to sulfites can also be related to genetic defects. In these cases, supplying the body with sulfur too quickly can overwhelm these pathways to result in symptoms like rashes both orally and on the skin. The solution to this is a slow dose increase and the addition of supportive nutrients to the pathway such as electrolytes including potassium (always take with food). Molybdenum and selenium assist the pathway. PQQ (pyrroloquinoline quinone) and Antioxidants decrease reactive oxygen species. Riboflavin helps to recycle sulfur-based glutathione.

23.6 HERX RESPONSES

A Herxheimer reaction, or Herx reaction for short, is the concept of getting worse before seeing improvement. Generally, it is a result of killing unwanted bacteria or yeast in the system and the body having to deal with the toxicity released from these organisms as they die.

We can also call this a *detox response*, as the body becomes temporarily overwhelmed by the toxicity of bacterial or yeast die-off until the liver detox pathways can upregulate to process it, or until the initial large quantity of die-off is reduced by treatment.

Herx reactions can be experienced as a flare in current symptoms or as acute symptoms like headaches or flu-like feelings of fatigue or achiness.[81]

I recommend gradual and incremental dose increase of GI Janel One to minimize Herx reactions, allowing these symptoms to gradually to resolve. Consider the Herx symptoms as part of a die-off response. In the long run you will be much more tolerant of dietary sulfur in foods.

I suspected that one of the reasons IBS/SIBO patients have so much trouble with higher sulfur foods is because the microbes are using the sulfur as their final electron receptor during anaerobic respiration and overwhelming the digestion with sulfur-based gases. The overgrowth of hydrogen sulfide-producing species contributes to this. The system cannot handle this high sulfur content all at once. However, follow the gradual titration with the GI Janel One treatment and, in the long run, you will have an easier time eating legumes, onions, garlic and raw cruciferous vegetables without gassy symptoms. I recommend waiting until you have completed your GI Janel One dosing before gradually adding back these foods.

23.7 FOOD SOURCES OF SULFUR

Since sulfur is found in amino acids, and amino acids are the building blocks of proteins, then protein foods are good dietary source of sulfur.

The sulfur-containing amino acids are methionine, taurine, homocysteine, cysteine and cystine. Eggs have a high amount of sulfur for feather production in the developing offspring. Meat, poultry, and fish also contain substantial amounts of sulfur.

Vegetables contain a different type of sulfur, called organosulfur. In vegan diets, sulfur is found in legumes, nuts and seeds. Sulfur is found in onions and garlic, the cruciferous vegetables (cabbage, cauliflower, broccoli, kale, collards and Brussels sprouts) and the radish family (turnips, radishes and daikon). Glutathione, the sulfur based nutrient and primary intercellular antioxidant that quenches damaging free radical formation can be found in radish and broccoli sprouts.

It's interesting to note that, just like the dosing of GI Janel One, these sulfur-rich foods need to be gradually ramped up in people with gas and bloating IBS/SIBO symptoms. I will usually suggest that a patient begin to slowly introduce these sulfur-rich foods like legumes and cruciferous vegetables once they have completed their full dosing schedule of GI Janel One. This typically goes very well. Sometimes I'll follow up with someone six to twelve months after completing their GI Janel protocol and they'll report a long list of these previously difficult-to-digest foods that they have successfully added back into their diet.

In general, sulfur-rich vegetables are not tolerated in large quantities prior to treatment with GI Janel One. Once the course of treatment is complete, they will be used to reacclimate the body to using the beneficial organosulfur compounds that they naturally provide. In this way, we are using food as medicine to continue the strengthening of the gastrointestinal barrier with organosulfur.

There are two B vitamins which contain sulfur: thiamin (vitamin B 1) and biotin (vitamin B7). Thiamin is found in organ meats, pork, whole grains, legumes, bran, and blackstrap molasses. Biotin is found in egg yolks, sardines, legumes, nuts, whole grains, cauliflower, mushrooms, and bananas.

23.8 Sulfur Deficiency and Toxicity

Organic sulfur has been overlooked in terms of deficiency states even though our soils are becoming more and more depleted of sulfur. This is likely because there is no known disorder directly associated with sulfur deficiency.

A deficiency of the structural action of sulfur can show up anywhere in the body from the microscopic cellular connections to the macroscopic connective tissue.

With a sulfur deficiency, the antioxidant properties of intracellular glutathione and the detoxification properties of glutathione conjugation lead to a myriad of symptom complexes rather than a specific diagnosis. This makes it less obvious that a sulfur-deficient state may be the primary cause, or one of the causes, of a diagnostic syndrome. Sulfur is the eighth most-concentrated element in the body, after oxygen, carbon, hydrogen, nitrogen, calcium, phosphorus, and potassium. It is the third most-concentrated mineral in the body.

The National Academy of Sciences (NAS) states no minimum or maximum requirement for sulfur in the diet. The NAS has little concern about either deficiency or toxicity. Deficiency occurs when the soil used for food growth is depleted of sulfur, when there is a deficiency of the proper intestinal bacteria, with low-protein diets, or with refined and highly processed diets.[82]

Animal studies were used to test long-term dosing of MSM. They found that levels of 1.5g/Kg resulted in no adverse events, mortality or gross physiological changes over 90 days of daily dosing. Applied to a 150-pound person, this would translate to a daily dose of 102 grams per day of MSM. Animal studies also found good absorption rates and excretion rates of MSM.[83][84]

I agree completely with Stephanie Seneff, PhD, a senior research scientist at MIT, who states that sulfate (sulfur) deficiency is the most common nutritional deficiency that you've never heard of.[85]

There are no known cautions for MSM, reasons to avoid it, or adverse interactions listed on the Epocrates Medical resource. [86]

23.9 THE CAUSE OF SULFUR DEPLETION

Essentially, it is the farming practices employing pesticides and chemicals meant to increase production that were introduced in the 1950's that have broken the sulfur cycle in food production. The cellular matrix study in 1999 investigated this concept to reveal that sulfur cycle plays a vital role in the regeneration of our cells. The study found that the use of chemical fertilizers had effectively broken the sulfur cycle in countries that use these fertilizers, lowering the sulfur content of crops. This effectively reduces the organosulfur available in our diets. [87]

23.10 SULFUR REQUIREMENTS

Sulfur is found in all plant and animal cells and comprises about 0.25% of your total body weight. There is no recommended daily intake for sulfur, but it is suggested by the National Academies Food and Nutrition Board to intake 0.2 to 1.5 grams daily.

Sulfur is the eighth most-common element in the human body, about equal in abundance to potassium.

We do not store sulfur in our bodies and must therefore receive a constant daily supply. [88]

Sulfur is the chemical element that is found in sulfa drugs, sulfites and sulfates. Sulfur is an essential element and is in amino acids and other important molecules in the body. Sulfur is an essential element for all life.

There are cofactors in the body such as glutathione and thioredoxin that require sulfur. When two sulfurs are connected, they make what is called a *disulfide bond*. This disulfide bond is what provides the mechanical strength of collagen and keratin. Keratin is what makes your skin tough and waterproof. Keratin is also in hair and feathers, giving them tensile strength.

The sulfur in plants is an organosulfur compound.

It is impossible to have a sulfur allergy. You cannot survive without sulfur, and it is one of the predominant elements in our body, acting both structurally and functionally. Allergies and intolerances can develop to sulfite or sulfonamides, but not to sulfur or sulfates.

The body needs about 850 mg of sulfur a day. Most of this comes from the four amino acids, which contain sulfur, or from vegetable sources of organosulfur. Microbes in the soil "fix" sulfur into a form that the growing plants can utilize, much like nitrogen is "fixed" by microbes for plant growth.

The sulfur-containing amino acids cysteine, cystine and methionine are important for the structure and function of insulin (blood sugar regulation) and heparin (anti-coagulant). Cellular respiration requires sulfur (production of energy). Sulfur is also a component of glutathione, which is the major intracellular antioxidant (stops free-radical damage). The liver uses sulfur also in the form of glutathione conjugation to eliminate body toxicity (detox).

MSM is methylsulfonylmethane with the chemical formula $(CH_3)_2 SO_2$. It is a sulfur containing compound (sulfur is the element; a compound is made of elements). It is also known as organic sulfur.

It is found in plant sources like Brussels sprouts, cabbage, broccoli, cauliflower, radish, daikon, turnips, garlic, onions, asparagus, legumes, kale, nuts, seeds, legumes, and wheat germ. The quantity of sulfur in plant sources depends on the quantity in the soil where they are grown. This group of foods is not well tolerated *before* your GI Janel treatment. You may have been put on a special diet to avoid these foods and the symptoms they cause. After your GI Janel treatment, though, you will tolerate these foods much better, with fewer symptoms, especially the uncomfortable gas and bloating caused by the high fibers and high sulfur content of the foods.

Sulfur is also found in animal products like eggs, meat, poultry, milk, and fish.[89]

24 GI JANEL ONE DOSING OVERVIEW

If you begin to use GI Janel One and your symptoms worsen, or you get smelly gas that passes, this is exciting news! GI Janel One can eventually resolve your gas and bloating symptoms if you listen to your body and increase it very gradually. When the gas passes, it does not get trapped in the intestines and cause that cramping, bloating discomfort that is the hallmark of SIBO.

The sulfur in GI Janel One is what may make you have smelly gas as your body acclimates to the dosing level. This is not the same as the gas produced in classic SIBO, which is methane or hydrogen gas. The gas that is created when using GI Janel One is hydrogen sulfide, and it will pass through you easily rather than creating trapped, gassy bloating. This will occur as the microbiome rebalances and the intestinal structure strengthens.

GI Janel One alleviates your bloating while it is treating your IBS/SIBO. As you increase your dose, your body will increase in its ability to utilize the GI Janel One, the bacteria and yeast will shift in their population, and the gas will subside. Soon, you will be able to take a full dose daily with no gas symptoms at all. This is your goal.

Remember to wait before you go up in dosing until the gas or any other die-off (Herx) reactions have resolved. The gas is an indication of your need for repair and re-population of your microbiome, so you can use this as a guide.

The initial gas is produced as the GI Janel One anaerobically breaks down in the intestine. The gas stops when the cells regain their strength, the bacteria levels drop, and the beneficial bacteria have grown in number to handle the dose of GI Janel One.

Hydrogen sulfide acts as a cell-signaling molecule. Cell-signaling molecules govern the basic cellular activities and coordinate the cellular actions. The cellular response to signaling is development, tissue repair, immunity and homeostasis.[90]

For those people that take over a week to adjust to their incremental dose increase of GI Janel and are no longer gassy, congratulations! You are helping make some important changes inside your body. Go slowly and take your time. Remember that your goal in the end is to be able to eat your foods freely without symptoms. I encourage you to do the work now, to reap the long-term benefits to come.

Some people like to do their dosing at nighttime, especially at the time of a dose increase. This way, you can be on your own if you need to pass gas. For someone who has suffered with the trapped gas and bloating of SIBO/IBS, it can be a real relief to have the freedom to pass that gas out of your body.

Remember, that the smelly gas is a sign that you are providing repair elements, and of the balancing of bacterial/yeast populations. It may be unpleasant but well worth it in the long run on your journey to eating what you want without having IBS/SIBO symptoms.

Here's more good news! The higher your dose, the less acclimation time or Herxheimer reactions you will have. Typically, once you reach 2-3 tsp daily, you can begin to increase your dosing much faster. However, I implore you to listen to your body. Every body is different, just like every fingerprint is unique. You will have your own unique timing. This is not a race, but a beautiful, balanced, orchestration within you.

> *Here's a case illustrating the power of GI Janel One. A 21-year-old woman came to see me, after trying to resolve her digestive symptoms with a local clinic. She had done both the IgG and the functional stool tests, so we had that ready to work with. Even with the treatment they attempted, she complained about episodes of diarrhea that were so severe, they left her dehydrated and requiring IV fluids for rehydration. Between these episodes she would be constipated for up to three days. She had gas and bloating pain all day long but noticed that her reflux and cramping pains were improved when off the identified IgG foods.*

Her symptoms all began after antibiotics were given for acne. The antibiotics initiated a C difficile infection. Following this infection, she saw a gastroenterologist, who performed a pH monitor, gastric emptying studies, an endoscopy, and colonoscopy with biopsies. All were clear.

My first step was to simplify her supplement use. I started her on GI Janel Digest A and Janel One at a low initial dose. I asked her to stop taking the many other supplements she was on until we got her digestive symptoms under control. I also simplified her IgG diet and asked her to avoid only those foods that impact the digestion. For her this was cow dairy, wheat, citrus fruits, sugar, and whole eggs. I added back dairy products made from goat, sheep, coconut, soy and buffalo, eggs as an ingredient in foods, gluten (non-wheat), fish and coffee, and requested that she use my soft food diet.

Four weeks later, she reported lessening of diarrhea and a feeling of a sour stomach with the Digest A formula. I switched her to my gentler Digest C formula with meals. She noted that her gas and bloating were worse on her starting dose of GI Janel One, which I assured her was normal and a good sign that we would see improvement in the long run. I then requested that she gradually increase her GI Janel One formula in 1/8 tsp increments. When I saw her again in four weeks, she was at a 2.5 tsp dose of GI Janel One twice daily. This is almost at the 6 tsp daily goal dose. She reported that her bloating and gas had resolved once she reached a 3 tsp dose of GI Janel One, but she then she continued to increase as I directed to achieve a therapeutic level. She noticed that her bowels had begun to move regularly after meals, and her stools were formed.

I kept her on a maintenance dose of GI Janel One at that point and gave her a course of Diflucan antifungal to clean up the yeast that was identified initially in her functional stool sample. I typically wait until a patient has completed their course of GI Janel One and then finish up with an antifungal treatment as it is much more effective and long lasting, once the system is stronger. We also did *a course of food-allergy desensitization, and she was able to add sugar, citrus, whole eggs and cow dairy successfully back into her diet. Wheat continued to be an issue in the form of pure bread, but she could have wheat-based cake and pie with no problems.*

It is now four years from the initial treatment, and I see her occasionally for follow-up visits for hip pain or her cat allergies, but her digestive symptoms have never returned.

The GI Janel One formula is a powder that can be mixed with food or drinks. This includes water, juice, fruit sauce, smoothies, puddings or other foods. You can mix it in water and then chase it with something stronger like juice. You can add flavors like chocolate or syrup and honey or stevia as you like. The stronger the dose is, the saltier it will taste.

Start with a single dose (1/2 tsp), and gradually increase (or decrease) based on your sensitivity level.

The most sensitive GI patients can have a Herxheimer reaction (or Herx for short). This is a die-off reaction as the GI Janel One kills off bacteria and yeast and the microbiome shifts. It is also a detoxification reaction as the GI Janel One is up-regulating the detox systems in your body. A Herxheimer reaction is a good sign that in the long run, you will have remarkable results with the use of GI Janel One.

Symptoms of Herxheimer can be malaise, fatigue, body aches, headache, flu-like feelings, and increased gassiness (but not trapped gas, it will pass through you). It may also be an exacerbation of any previous symptoms you may have experienced.

As you continue with your dose increases, those unwanted symptoms should gradually resolve completely, and the original IBS/SIBO symptoms of gas, bloating and abdominal pain will diminish.

Each time you increase your dose of GI Janel One, some of the symptoms may occur again but to a lessened extent. When you get to the higher doses (2-3 teaspoons and above) where the digestive system will be stronger, you can increase easily, without the experience of a Herxheimer reaction or gassiness.

People who have a CBS (cystathionine beta-synthase enzyme) defect in their methylation pathways may have a metabolic backup or may kick off more irritants as their bodies utilize the GI Janel One. This can manifest as body aches, as a temporary rash or an exacerbation of aphthous ulcers (canker sores). This defect can be detected using genetic testing, which is available online. A longer, slower dose increase is recommended if you have this defect. You will not need to escalate to the full dose.

25 GI JANEL ONE, DOSING SPECIFICS

For many people, you'll want to go through the steps that I have outlined and remove any offending foods (See the Diet chapter), then begin your GI Janel digestive supplements as your first step in treatment.

If your primary symptoms are uncomfortable gas and bloating regardless of what you eat or drink, put yourself on the fast track and *start* with GI Janel One as I recommend in the "Fast Track" Chapter. Starting the fast track, you may save time and eliminate all the extra work of removing foods from your diet. What have you got to lose? You're already uncomfortable.

For people with IBS/SIBO-D (diarrhea), IBS/SIBO-M (diarrhea and constipation), or with colitis, I recommend beginning GI Janel One as I have traditionally recommended. This means you must first remove the intolerant foods. What I have seen in practice is that once you are on a moderate dose of GI Janel One (2-3 tsp per day), if foods sneak into your diet that previously had caused symptoms, the body is less reactive or even symptom free. I have seen this even with Crohn's patients!

People with IBS/SIBO-C (constipation) will need to get their bowels moving using GI Janel AM/BM prior to the use of GI Janel One.

25.1 FORMULA MIXING IDEAS

Mix GI Janel One in one to four ounces of juice or water and add any of the following to taste.

- Naturally or artificially flavored syrup
- Honey
- Maple syrup
- Stevia
- Coconut sugar
- Monk Fruit

You can also use it plain water first, then chase it with a flavor or juice you enjoy.

You can add it to fruit sauce, puddings, smoothies or any other food you would like to try that you know you tolerate. Smoothies disguise the flavor well in the lower doses.

25.2 DOSING LEVELS

25.2.1 The very delicate patient

•   Start with a tiny pinch of GI Janel One. Continue at this level for four weeks, or until taking the formula causes no Herxheimer or adverse symptoms,

•   Then, increase your dose to 1/8 of a teaspoon daily for 2 weeks, or until the formula causes no Herxheimer symptoms. You may have to increase slowly, by one pinch at a time, to reach this goal.

•   Then increase the dose to ½ tsp daily for two weeks, or until the formula causes no Herx symptoms. You may have to slowly get to this ½ tsp goal using one pinch at a time increases.

•   Now you can likely increase the dose more quickly as Herx reactions will be less. Increase by ¼- ½ teaspoon each 3-7 days as tolerated, working your way up to the goal dose.

•   Your goal dose is 2 heaping tablespoons a day (6 heaping teaspoons) for 60 days. This can be taken in divided doses throughout the day or a single dose (it will taste strong). An example of a divided dose would be 2 heaping teaspoons three times daily.

I have had patients who are only able to increase the GI Janel One dosing by pinch increments, even after they are above the 1 teaspoon dose. This is rare. The outcome is the same as in a stronger patient, however. Eventually around the 1-2 teaspoon dose, they stop having the daily gas and bloating pain or distention.

25.2.2 The moderately sensitive patient

•   Start with 1/8 of a teaspoon of GI Janel One, daily for 1-2 weeks until any Herx symptoms to abate. (You may not have any Herx reactions.)

•   Then increase to ½ teaspoon of GI Janel daily for 1-2 weeks, until any Herx symptoms abate.

•   Then you can increase the GI Janel One formula each 3-7 days by ½ tsp, again waiting for any Herx symptoms or increased gassiness to abate.

•   Your goal dose is 2 heaping tablespoons a day (6 heaping teaspoons) for 60 days. This can be taken in divided doses throughout the day or a single dose (it will taste strong). An example of a divided dose would be 2 heaping teaspoons three times daily.

25.2.3 The strong patient

•   Start with 1/8 tsp of GI Janel daily. You should have no Herx reactions or gas increase. If you do, then drop down to the moderate sensitivity dosing recommendations.

•   Begin to increase your dose by 1 tsp each 1-5 days. You should have no Herx reactions, although your stools may change (loose or firmer depending on your type of IBS/SIBO). This is expected; just let your body get acclimated before jumping to the next dose level.

•   You will quickly get to the treatment dose of 2 heaping tablespoons a day (6 heaping teaspoons) and hold it there for 60 days. This can be taken in divided doses or all at once. An example of a divided dose would be 2 heaping teaspoons three times daily.

Caveat: You thought you were a strong or moderate responder, but are having Herx symptoms

•   Slow down!

•   Go back to your previous dose level. If you are just starting treatment, go back to a tiny pinch of the formula and keep it there until your Herx symptoms abate. Trust me, this is a very positive indication that eventually you will have symptom relief. Everyone is different, so don't compare your progress to someone else. Be patient with yourself. The Herx symptoms are a positive sign that you will eventually get rid of your symptoms at the higher doses of GI Janel One.

25.2.4   The Fast Track

I recommend this treatment for patients who experience their gas, bloating and cramping no matter what they eat, drink or even if they don't eat at all.

For the fast track you do not have to make any dietary changes. You do not need to take any extra digestive supplements. If you are constipated, get your bowels moving first by taking GI Janel AM / BM. Once your bowels are moving daily, then begin your dosing of GI Janel One. You can use any of the dosing frequencies that I have listed above.

It's as simple as that. That's all you need to do.

26 THE GI JANEL FAMILY

26.1 GI JANEL DIGEST A

GI Janel Digest A supports the initial phase of digestion, which occurs in the stomach. The healthy stomach is like a strong, flexible, hollow ball. During digestion, this ball is filled with acid. The acid is extremely important and accomplishes several key aspects of digestion.

During digestion, stomach acid can get as low as a pH of 1. This is the pH level of battery acid! There are many reasons that this acid level is important.

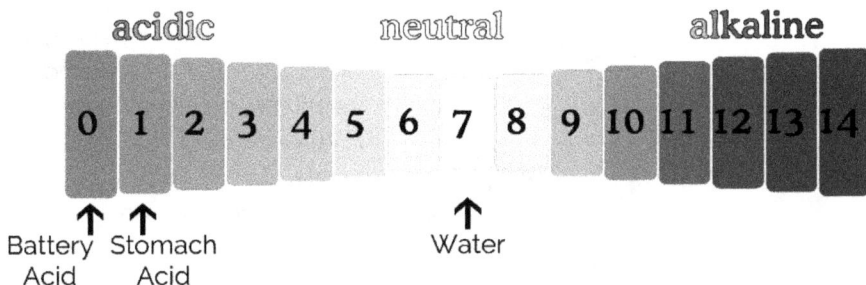

Figure 26.1 The pH of the stomach

First, the enzymes that begin the breakdown of proteins in your food work best in this acidic environment.

Second, the acidity protects us by killing some of the bacteria, yeast and other pathogens that we ingest with our food. You can imagine how important this is for SIBO patients. You don't want to be adding to the bacteria or yeast in your small intestines with your meals.

Remember our food is not sterile! We need many protective features throughout the digestive track to ensure that we don't get sick from the critters that come in with the food we eat. I refer you back to the earlier chapter on LGS and the gastrointestinal barrier.

For IBS/SIBO relief, adequate stomach acidity (if tolerated) is imperative! If there is not enough acid in the stomach, food will not be broken down properly right from the beginning. This leaves food particles that can feed bacteria, increasing bacteria overgrowth. This causes increased gas and pressure in the abdomen, which even can impact reflux! (The gas can push upwards.) If hydrogen sulfide-producing species are predominant in the upper GI, this gas can feel hot like heartburn. One ounce of carbohydrates that is undigested could produce more than ten quarts of hydrogen gas in the small intestine. Ouch.

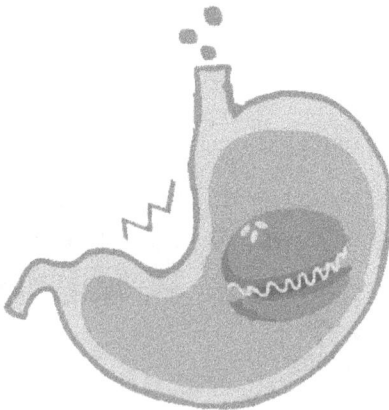

Figure 26.2 *Low stomach acid leaves undigested food particles. Undigested food particles feed bacteria and yeast, promoting their growth. Overgrowth of bacterial and yeast species produce gas which increases pressure that is experienced as bloating or even reflux.*

Thirdly, the acidity in the stomach is necessary to begin the process required for vitamin B12 and mineral absorption. Therefore, people on acid blockers can get more infections, are more prone to osteoporosis (weakened bones), and can have much lower levels of B12, which results in fatigue.

There is some information emerging about the increase in stomach cancers for people using long term acid blockers after H pylori infections have been treated. We believe that the killing of upper GI bacteria, using the triple therapy, followed by acid suppression can wreak havoc on the immune/microbial relationship in the system.[91]

I begin treatment of IBS/SIBO with the GI Janel Digest A supplement because it is a perfect clinical trial to determine the strength of the stomach lining.

Remember, *the pH of the stomach secretions can be as strong as battery acid*. Since these secretions are very acidic, we need to have a lot of protection in the lining of the stomach so that we don't burn a hole right through it (this is what an ulcer is). This protection is in the form of a mucous layer.

If you take the GI Janel Digest A and feel a burning or GERD (gastrointestinal reflux or heartburn), then you are either producing hyperchlorhydria (high stomach acid secretion), which is rare especially in IBS/SIBO, or the protective lining of your stomach is not strong enough to contact normal acidity. This is much more common. If this occurs, then there will need to be a lot of healing of the stomach lining as a part of your protocol. Remember from previous chapters that acidity is needed to keep the valve between the stomach and esophagus closed tight. It's counterintuitive but adding acidity for people having reflux can be the answer to stopping the reflux symptoms if the tissue layers and mucous layers have not been compromised.

On the other hand, if you take the GI Janel Digest A and do not experience burning or GERD, then keep taking it with your meals. You are replacing the initial phase of digestion, which triggers the subsequent phases as your food moves through the digestive system. You are improving your ability to absorb minerals and B12, and you are improving your protection from infection. You are also upregulating the gastro colic reflex and improving motility.[92] [93 94 95 96 97]

GI Janel Digest A contains Betaine HCL (750 mg) and pepsin (50 mg). Pepsin is the first step of protein digestion in the stomach. Pepsin is activated at the low pH provided by Betaine HCL.

GI Janel Digest A improves the activation and absorption of B12, minerals (like calcium) and protects you from infections by killing pathogens (bacteria, viruses) that are ingested with food. Use 1-4 capsules before meals to decrease gas and bloating, constipation or fullness after eating small amounts.

Do not use the product if you have been diagnosed with active gastritis or ulcers or if the use of it causes burning or worsens reflux. Gi Janel Digest A is Non-GMO.

26.2 GI JANEL DIGEST B

GI Janel Digest B is the most comprehensive of the GI Janel Digestion formulas. This is because it is formulated to support the gastric (stomach), the pancreatic, the gall bladder, and the intestinal cell phases of digestion.

GI Janel Digest B will support the acidic phase of digestion, which occurs in the stomach. This is like what GI Janel Digest A does. In addition, GI Janel Digest B contains digestive enzymes that work at a higher pH. These digestive enzymes are often deficient or reduced in cases of IBS/SIBO, and for some people, the addition of this support is all they need to eliminate their symptoms. This is typically the case in Exocrine Pancreatic Insufficiency or EPI.

Most everyone has heard of the well-known enzyme deficiency *lactose intolerance*. This is a specific deficiency of an enzyme that is produced in the lining of the small intestinal cells. This enzyme is called lactase and it functions to break down the sugar called lactose which is found in milk products.

There are other enzyme deficiencies present in SIBO/IBS that make the breakdown of carbohydrates, fats and proteins inefficient. This leads to symptoms. GI Janel Digest B supports the breakdown of all these food macromolecules, allowing you to fully digest carbohydrates, fats and proteins. This will not only decrease symptoms of gas, bloating and abdominal pain, but it will enable your body to absorb these food nutrients more effectively and take some digestive stress off your system.

Begin your IBS/SIBO relief by taking one of the GI Janel Digestive formulas at your meals and snacks. If your symptoms improve, then continue using your GI Janel Digest supplements through the protocol. This will support the digestive process and allow your body to go back into homeostasis (its natural balanced state). GI Janel Digest formulas can even eliminate unwanted bacteria or yeasts by making the environment hospitable again to digestion, rather than to the overgrowth of bacteria or yeasts.

As the lining of your intestine heals with the GI Janel protocols, the environment will again become accommodating to the production of intestinal enzymes. This will mean an increased ability to breakdown carbohydrates. Then guess what? Your carbohydrate intolerance and lactose intolerance can improve or resolve. Of course, this is unless you have genetically based lactose intolerance or other carbohydrate intolerance.

The third component of GI Janel Digest B is bile, which supports the breakdown of fats. Anyone who has had their gall bladder removed will benefit from taking supplemental bile with meals. If SIBO/IBS patients are having chronic diarrhea or gas due to fat malabsorption, taking ox bile to increase fat absorption is a simple step to improve or relieve these symptoms.

In summary, if you cannot tolerate the acidity of GI Janel Digest A and you get heartburn when you use it, then move to GI Janel Digest B. If this improves your symptoms, continue to use it with meals. If you cannot tolerate the acidity of GI Janel Digest A or B, then move onto GI Janel Digest C.

GI Janel Digest B supports the digestion of proteins, fats and carbohydrates.

Use 1-2 capsules before meals to decrease gas and bloating, constipation or fullness after eating. GI Janel Digest B also activates protein digestion in the stomach with betaine HCL. This formula contains DDP IV (dipeptidyl peptidase IV) which breaks down the casomorphin in dairy (casein) and gluteomorphin (in gluten). The lactase enzyme in GI Janel Digest B aids in the breakdown of lactose (dairy sugar).

Do not use this product if you have been diagnosed with active gastritis or ulcers or if the use causes burning or the worsening of reflux.

26.3 GI JANEL DIGEST C

GI Janel Digest C is the gentlest of the digest formulas. It supports the pancreatic phase of digestion. It is plant-based, and therefore suitable for vegetarian or vegan diets.

Once the food has left the stomach, it enters the small intestine where it continues to be digested by pancreatic enzymes. These enzymes are made in the exocrine pancreas. They travel through a tube that leads from the pancreas to the small intestine. As the food makes its way through the 25 feet of small intestine, it is broken into smaller and smaller particles by the digestive enzymes. Once the food reaches the second half of the small intestine, it is transported microscopically and moves from the intestine and into the body.

Unless there is damage in the esophagus, stomach or small intestine, taking GI Janel Digest C should be soothing and helpful for digestive issues such as bloating or digestive pain. If there is any inflammation in any of these systems, then even this gentle formula can cause you to feel more heartburn. In this case, the healing phase must be pursued and completed before digestion can be assisted by the GI Janel Digest formulas.

GI Janel Digest C is a gentle digestive support to improve the breakdown and absorption of carbohydrates, proteins and fats in the diet. Use this formula with meals for gas, bloating, irregularity, or a feeling of fullness after eating.

Do not use if you have been diagnosed with active ulcers or gastritis. Discontinue use if reflux worsens. Made with non-GMO ingredient, suitable for vegetarian and vegan diets.

26.4 GI Jan-Aloe

GI Jan-Aloe is truly a healing tour de force. It is the most powerful formula that I've used to regenerate the mucous protection of the intestinal wall.

It's a very simple supplement, and that is what the digestion likes: simplicity. It takes 200 pounds of aloe vera inner gel fillets to make one pound of this nourishing aloe extract. This means that each time you take one capsule of GI Jan-Aloe, you are introducing the soothing and healing properties of an enormous quantity of aloe plant.

The outside of the aloe plant (dark green) has laxative properties. This part of the plant is contraindicated in pregnancy and lactation. This outer layer is not included in GI Jan-Aloe. GI Jan-Aloe is pure inner aloe gel fillet, which contains concentrated mucilaginous polysaccharides to soothe and heal.

This has become my go-to product for hyperacidity and reflux so that my patients can heal and get off their reflux medications. It is also one of the primary supplements that I use to repair the intestine and soothe tummy pain. As a bonus, Aloe mucopolysaccharides are immune-stimulating, so you may find that when you're taking it to repair leaky gut or heartburn, your immune defenses are stronger, and you are less vulnerable to cold and flu viruses.

GI Jan-Aloe is the strongest, natural healing supplement that I have come across in 20 years. It is unparalleled in resolving the symptoms of heartburn and healing the intestinal wall.

The phytonutrients in GI Jan-Aloe are never heated above 99° Fahrenheit and are not highly processed. This ensures a product that retains the strong healing properties of the plant. The long polysaccharide chains remain intact in the same way they are found in nature.

Using GI Jan-Aloe to heal the digestive tract and to relieve heartburn can stimulate the immune system. With the gentle preparation of this supplement, the natural Aloe polysaccharide chains remain intact. The longer the polysaccharide chain of the aloe phytonutrients, the greater the effectiveness in supporting immune and healing function. Gi Jan-Aloe is non-GMO.

26.5 GI JANEL ONE

GI Janel One is my flagship supplement and is what makes the GI Janel system unique. This is the treatment that is targeted to resolve the gas and bloating common in IBS and SIBO. GI Janel One can be used as a standalone treatment or can be combined with other GI Janel supplements.

In addition to alleviating the symptoms of gas and bloating, GI Janel One provides the raw substance for healing the connective tissue of the bowels, and thus restores the gastrointestinal barrier. As part of the cellular regeneration, motility is also improved. GI Janel One acts as a natural antibiotic and antifungal, and it will help the bowels to move more regularly for both diarrhea and constipation.

GI Janel One contains methylsulfonylmethane and acacia fiber. Acacia is the preferred fiber for IBS and SIBO treatment. It is a very gentle soluble fiber derived from the acacia plant. GI Janel One is also formulated with soothing and protective marshmallow root and slippery elm herbs.

You will find more extensive information on GI Janel One in a previous chapter, including dosing and the research and science behind this powerful IBS/SIBO formulation.

26.6 GI JANEL AM / BM

GI Janel AM / BM is formulated to improve bowel motility and tone. It contains magnesium hydroxide as a mild, osmotic laxative. It also contains Triphala from fruit, which has been used for centuries in classic Ayurvedic medicine (the traditional medicine of India).

Triphala is a blend of three fruits: Amla (*Emblica officinalis*), chebulic myrobalan (*Terminalia chebula*), and Belleric myrobalan (*Terminalia belerica*). This blend is anti-inflammatory and has antioxidant properties.

Indian Gooseberry, also known as Amla, is responsible for the detoxification effect. It is rich in vitamin C. Amla reduces inflammation in the digestive system and acts as a mild laxative. It is gentle for people with very sensitive digestive systems.

Belleric myrobalan helps with body detoxification by specifically clearing unproductive mucous congestion. It is a strong astringent like the other myrobalan, which supports tone and strength.

Chebulic myrobalan has antioxidant properties which can help to protect and support the body. Also called Haritaki, this plant contains mild laxatives known as anthraquinone phytonutrients. The high tannin content is astringent and helps to tonify and strengthen the digestive lining. This supports effective peristalsis and provides protection against prolapse, ulcerations, and gastrointestinal barrier defects. It is traditionally believed to have some antimicrobial properties for parasitic or other infections.

GI Janel AM / BM can be used for occasional constipation, or daily as a bowel tonic to strengthen and tonify the digestive system. GI Janel AM/BM is Non-GMO.

27 Symptom and Treatment

In this chapter, I hope to provide you with a clear guide to manage your GI Janel treatment. Please find the symptoms that match yours and follow the protocol I outlined. Before beginning treatment, it is important that you rule out any urgent and critical reasons for your symptoms with your doctor.

27.1 Bloating Distention / SIBO

Bloating distention with no other GI symptoms is the *classic* and possibly standalone SIBO/SIFO symptom. If you have constant abdominal distention without diarrhea or constipation and without any abdominal pain or reflux, then you may indeed simply have an overgrowth of bacterial species in your small intestine. The following are your treatment steps. Stop your treatment and hold it at the step that resolves your symptoms. Complete your GI Janel One dosing to heal and strengthen the system.

Step one:

- Take one or two capsules of GI Janel Digest A, B or C formula with each meal. Start with GI Janel Digest A. If tolerated, you can take up to six capsules of GI Janel Digest A with meals. If you experience any heartburn from taking one capsule of GI Janel Digest A, then stop and move to GI Janel Digest B. If you experience heartburn from this, then stop and move to GI Janel Digest C. If you know that you are sensitive, start with GI Janel Digest C.

Step two:

- Use a soft food diet and Identify and remove food triggers (see chapters on the soft food diet. It may be helpful to eat a diet that removes all grain-based carbohydrates until finished with your GI Janel One dosing. This is basically a paleo diet, but it is okay to eat high density vegetable carbohydrates like potatoes.

Step three:

- Use the doses described in the section on GI Janel One and follow the protocol to the 6 heaping teaspoons as your full dose. Most people will have symptoms alleviated once they reach the therapeutic dose. If bloating/distention is not completely resolved, then do a final sweep with antimicrobial/fungal therapy. Continue your full 8 weeks of the therapeutic dose of GI Janel One with your antimicrobial therapy.

- My preference for antimicrobial therapy is a combination of berberine (Hydrastis) and oils (thyme, clove, rosemary and oregano). Also helpful are: garlic, caprylic acid, and undecylenic acid. Various herbal parasitic formulas can also be added. These include herbs like gentian and wormwood.

27.2 ABDOMINAL PAIN, NON-GASSY

Move through these steps and stop at the level where your symptoms resolve. This will be different for each person due to the degree of the underlying cause of your IBS/SIBO, the individual complexity, and the degree of microscopic damage to your gastrointestinal barrier.

Step one:

- Take one or two capsules of GI Janel Digest A, B or C formula with each meal. Start with GI Janel Digest A. If tolerated, you can take up to six capsules of GI Janel Digest A with meals. If you experience any heartburn from taking one capsule of GI Janel Digest A, then stop and move to GI Janel Digest B. If you experience heartburn from this, then stop and move to GI Janel Digest C. If you know that you are sensitive, start with GI Janel Digest C.

Step two:

- Take one capsule of GI Jan-Aloe daily and as needed for pain or reflux.

Step three:

- Ensure that your bowels are moving every day and that you feel a full evacuation after moving your bowels. (See constipation treatment.)

Step four:

- Use a soft food diet and Identify and remove food triggers. (See the chapters on the soft food diet.)

Step five:

- Begin dosing GI Janel One, gradually increasing your dose as tolerated. Your final dose will be 1 tablespoon (3 teaspoons) all at once, or in divided doses daily. (Use the doses described in the section on GI Janel One.)

Step six:

- Identify and remove any digestive bacterial, yeast or parasite growths. (See the section on functional stool testing.)

27.2.1 Differential Diagnosis

Below are the causes of acute or chronic abdominal pain. These must be ruled out or identified prior to proceeding with a function approach to IBS/SIBO treatment.

27.2.1.1 *Digestive Tract*
- Gastro esophageal reflux disease (GERD)
- Peptic or gastric ulcer
- Crohn's disease / ulcerative colitis (IBD)
- Collagenous, lymphocytic, eosinophilic colitis
- Infectious gastroenteritis
- Intestinal obstruction
- Celiac disease
- Lactose intolerance

27.2.1.2 *Digestive Organs*
- Pancreatitis
- Gall stones or gall bladder inflammation

27.2.1.3 *Cancers*
- Esophageal cancer
- Gastric (stomach) cancer
- Colorectal cancer
- Liver cancer
- Pancreatic cancer
- Cholangiocarcinoma

27.2.1.4 *Kidney disease*
- Kidney stones
- Chronic kidney infection

27.2.1.5 *Reproductive disease*
- Endometriosis
- Uterine fibroids
- Pelvic inflammatory disease
- Ovarian cysts

27.2.1.6 *Neurological disease*
- Gastroparesis (delayed emptying of the stomach into the small intestine)
- Dyspepsia
- Narcotic bowel syndrome
- Abdominal migraine
- Centrally mediated abdominal pain syndrome
- Chronic abdominal wall pain

27.2.1.7 *Systemic disease*
- Heavy metal poisoning (lead, arsenic)
- Myotoxicity
- Familial Mediterranean fever
- Acute intermittent porphyria
- Paroxysmal nocturnal hemoglobinuria

27.2.1.8 *Vessel disease*
- Chronic mesenteric ischemia (loss of blood flow)
- Superior mesenteric artery syndrome

27.2.1.9 *Referred pain*
- Pain coming from another system in the body

27.3 ABDOMINAL PAIN, GASSY (SIBO/SIFO)

Step one:

- Take one or two capsules of GI Janel Digest A, B or C formula with each meal. Start with GI Janel Digest A. If tolerated, you can take up to six capsules of GI Janel Digest A with meals. If you experience any heartburn from taking one capsule of GI Janel Digest A, then stop and move to GI Janel Digest B. If you experience heartburn from this, then stop and move to GI Janel Digest C. If you know that you are sensitive, start with GI Janel Digest C.

Step two:

- Take One GI Jan-Aloe daily and as needed for pain or reflux

Step three:

- Ensure that your bowels are moving every day and that you feel fully evacuated (see constipation)

Step four:

- Use the soft food diet and Identify and remove food triggers (see diet chapters)

Step five:

- If gas and bloating persist regardless of the type of food you eat, you likely have SIBO/SIFO, or large intestinal dysbiosis, and need to follow the GI Janel One Protocol. (See the chapter on dosing for GI Janel One.)

27.3.1 Differential Diagnosis

Gas pain is associated with the following symptoms: voluntary or involuntary passing of gas (burping or flatus), a knotted feeling in the abdominal area, abdominal swelling or tightness, a sensation that clothes get tighter, or sharp pains or cramps that occur anywhere in abdomen and that change locations quickly or resolve quickly. These pains can be very intense. It is normal to pass gas 10-20 times a day depending on your diet.

The disorders to be ruled out are:

- Gallstones
- Heart disease
- Appendicitis
- Ovarian Cancer

You should see your doctor for these symptoms:

Blood in your stool, changes in stool color or frequency, chronic abdominal pain, unusual weight changes, chest pain and persistent nausea or vomiting.

27.4 CONSTIPATION

Before we get started with treatment, let me tell you about a case that represents many patients with constipation and SIBO whom I have treated over the years.

> A fifty-year-old female, who had been living with her symptoms for decades, had already seen her gastroenterologist and had a colonoscopy and endoscopy. Since these were completely normal scopes, her symptoms were clearly functional. She complained of years of constipation. She would move her bowels only once each seven to fourteen days. Occasionally she would take the herb cascara to relieve her constipation. She had bloating pain which started around noon every day and diminished overnight. She noticed that her constipation and bloating pain were worse when she ate

cow dairy, so she avoided those foods. In an attempt to alleviate her symptoms, she had previously had her gall bladder removed, but nothing changed following this surgery. I immediately put her on my soft food diet, and began her on GI Janel Digest A with her meals to get motility started and kill some overgrowth. I also had her do a supervised magnesium flush, so I could assess the degree of treatment required to get her bowels moving daily. She began this while we waited for her IgG results.

When she returned, she reported that after taking two capsules of magnesium oxide (400 mg per capsule) every two hours, she required a total of eighteen capsules on a Saturday to get some hard rocks of stools to move out on the following day. She repeated this dose and her stools began to move more softly, a little each day. We halved the dose to nine capsules of magnesium oxide, divided throughout the day and she continued this. Following the magnesium flush, she told me that her bloating pain was better, and she was less gassy overall. Her IgG testing was positive for cow dairy, goat dairy, whole eggs, soy and gluten. Those are the GI significant reactions that I asked her to eliminate and challenge prior to her next visit. The other reactions that were IgG positive were almond, lentils, oat, peas, peanut, and cranberry. I did not ask her to avoid these. I saw her again in six weeks and by removing the IgG foods (she decided to just keep them all out of her diet, rather than challenge each food), we were able to cut back on her magnesium dosing. The reason for this is that by eliminating the inflammation caused by the foods, the magnesium was able to work more effectively.

At that point, I switched her to GI Janel AM/BM so that she could have the impact of the magnesium hydroxide in addition to bulking for her stools. I added in the GI Janel One and she began her gradual dose increase. Once she achieved the three-teaspoon dose of GI Janel One, she reported daily formed stools and no abdominal pain or bloating. She did become gassier when dosing the GI Janel One, so she would take it at nighttime in order to pass the gas while she slept.

Once she reached her full dose of six teaspoons of GI Janel One and had maintained it for eight weeks, I cut her down to a maintenance dose. She began to add her IgG foods back into her diet and found that now, only dairy or too much sugar made her gassy. She kept these out of her diet. She really wanted to start eating cruciferous vegetables again, so we started with well-cooked versions and gradually brought these back into her diet. By the time I saw her again four months later, she was able to eat raw cauliflower and broccoli without a problem. This was years ago now. I continue to see her for her annual lab work and menopause management. Her digestive symptoms have never returned.

Before you do anything else, get your bowels moving! Your bowels are one of the major detoxification systems for your entire body. If waste sits around in them, you are potentially re-absorbing chemicals that your body is trying to get rid of through your stool. The term for this is *enterohepatic recirculation.*

Chronic constipation results in gassiness and abdominal pain that must be addressed prior to the initiation of other treatments. Once you have started your GI Janel Digest formula (A, B or C), if you still have constipation, then continue with the information below.

Your bowels need to move every day. It takes 12-24 hours for a healthy digestive tract to extract the nutrition from your food and move it through your body.

In a healthy system, one meal is being eaten while the previous meal is moving from the small intestine to the large (all nutrients extracted). The food consumed two meals ago is waiting to exit the rectum.

When you eat, there is a reflex that signals the release of stool from your body. This is called the *gastrocolic reflex* and it is caused by the food stretching your stomach and the byproducts of digestion entering your small intestine from the stomach. With a healthy system, it is possible to have a bowel movement after every meal. In indigenous cultures where the food has not been overly processed and refined, bowel movements can typically occur three times a day, one after each meal.

I am happy if my patients can move their bowels once daily. In cases of chronic constipation, this is my initial goal.

How to reave up a slow, sluggish digestive system? Start from the top.

Step one:

- Take one or two capsules of GI Janel Digest A, B or C formula with each meal. Start with GI Janel Digest A. If tolerated, you can take up to six capsules of GI Janel Digest A with meals. If you experience any heartburn from taking one capsule of GI Janel Digest A, then stop and move to GI Janel Digest B. If you experience heartburn from this, then stop and move to GI Janel Digest C. If you know that you are sensitive, start with GI Janel Digest C.

Continue your digest supplements as you move to step two. They are building the foundation for your body to eventually move on its own

Step two:

GI Janel AM/BM

- Take two capsules, twice daily.

- This is where things become very individualized. Too much will loosen the stools and cause diarrhea. This is not necessarily a terrible thing as you'll certainly need to cleanse out the bowels at some level. Adjust your dose to what works for you and hold it there. This might be as high as two to four capsules, three times a day. There can be a three to five-day delay as the GI Janel AM/BM begins to build so adjust gradually in either direction, whether dosing up or down.

- You can start with two capsules twice daily for five days. If your bowels have not moved in five days, then increase to five capsules a day for another five days. Continue to increase each five days by one additional capsule until your bowels move. What you are looking for is one to three soft bowel movements a day.

- Start by getting your bowels moving, even if they are loose, then reduce the dose by one capsule very slowly, every five days until the dose is moving your bowels one to three times a day (even if it is a loose movement). Stop there and hold your dose constant. It may take three to five days for your bowels to adjust in either direction.

- Once your bowels start moving, hold your dosing constant. If you reduce the dose, be sure to gradually decrease by one capsule no more often than each five days. If you're having stools more frequently than three times a day, then decrease your dose in this same, gradual manner by one capsule each five days. Ensure that you are drinking plenty of water to replace the water you are losing with loose stools.

- There can be a delayed reaction as the dosing builds up or down, so a gradual increase or decrease is the key here.

- If your bowels stop after three to five days as your dose decreases, then increase back to the level where they previously moved and hold it there.

- If after five days of dosing GI Janel AM/BM at 12 capsules per day, your bowels are not moving then see you provider about a magnesium or vitamin C flush.

Step three:

Once you've found the dose of GI Janel AM/BM that works for you, keep it consistent every day. At this point you can begin to add in your GI Janel One. Once you have your bowels moving with GI Janel AM/BM and you add in the GI Janel One, it will eventually take over the job. Most people can slowly decrease and discontinue the dose of GI Janel AM/BM.

Start your GI Janel One dose slowly with ½ tsp and increase by ½ tsp each three to five days. If your bowels slow down, then hold your dose until they start to move again. Continue to increase your GI Janel One dose gradually to the therapeutic dose of one or two heaping tablespoons a day (This is equivalent to 3 to 6 heaping teaspoons). As you increase your GI Janel One, your bowels should become formed and full, and you will be detoxing nicely. At this time, you can start to decrease GI Janel AM/BM and let the GI Janel One take care of moving your bowels.

More information for using the GI Janel One supplement can be found in the chapters on GI Janel One.

It is important to be consuming between 40-70 ounces of filtered water or other non- caffeinated beverages daily. You can use herbal punches or teas, diluted juice, electrolyte tablets, Recharge or other healthy choices for your fluid intake. Caffeinated and alcoholic beverages are diuretics, and count against your fluid intake.

It can be helpful to stretch your sigmoid colon using a stool or a squatty-potty. This will elevate your legs and put your body in a squatting position for bowel movements. This is extremely helpful for people who have had long term constipation that has resulted in a rectocele (loss of elastic recoil and outpouching of the colon). For these people, putting pressure on the perineum (above the rectum and below the reproductive organs) can be helpful when having a bowel movement.

Another therapy used in Ayurveda (ancient Indian medicine) is to drink a cup of hot water with the juice of one-half to a whole lemon each morning, 30-to-60 minutes before eating. This can be helpful to initiate bowel movements and to train the bowels to move in the morning. Lemon contains the phytochemical D-Limonene which is helpful for GI motility. Coffee (if tolerated) can also stimulate bowel movements.

Constipation responds well to coffee enemas, and this can also improve bile secretion for digestion and can improve glutathione levels. Check with your physician prior to using coffee enemas, as there can be adverse reactions if they are inappropriate for you.

Once you get your bowels moving, the basics to avoid constipation returning are water, exercise, and fiber in the diet. In IBS/SIBO, the preferential fiber is gentle, water soluble fiber (see the section on diet). GI Janel One contains the best type of soluble fiber for IBS/SIBO, as it is very low fermenting. I have some patients use GI Janel One as a long-term support even after the chronic IBS/SIBO symptoms have resolved. This will continue to supply your body with sulfur for structural maintenance of the digestive system.

27.4.1 Constipation is not a laxative deficiency... but

MiraLAX (polyethylene glycol 3550) certainly lacks the added health benefits that you will get from using GI Janel AM/BM or magnesium. However, it may be easier to use and may get your bowels moving equally well, so that is an option if you choose.

Polyethylene glycol (PEG) is an osmotic laxative. This means that it draws water into the intestines so that stools are less dry. As a result, they can be bulkier and more frequent. Use as directed and talk to your doctor if your bowels have not moved after seven days of proper use.

Do not use polyethylene glycol if you have any allergy to it, or it affects the efficacy of any other medications that you are on. Talk to your doctor prior to initiating treatments. PEG is recommended for occasional constipation so once your bowels start to move, you may want to switch over to GI Janel AM/BM and GI Janel One as outlined in the previous section.

Long-term use of polyethylene glycol can result in chronic constipation as your bowels become dependent on it to move. This is not the case with GI Janel AM/BM or GI Janel One. They are providing the smooth muscles of your intestines with what they need so they can regain their normal peristaltic movement and eventually work well on their own. The digestion can regain function if the rest of the system has been repaired and offending foods removed from the diet for the healing period.

The MiraLAX website and Web MD have good summaries for the use and precautions around the use of polyethylene glycol.

Absorption is less than 2%, which is good because this chemical is used as a chemical solvent, so it's probably not something you want absorbing into your body with long-term use. The smaller the body, the faster that concentration can make an impact.

The CDC has nasty list of adverse effects and toxicity caused by ethylene glycol. If you string many ethylene glycols together, you end up with "many ethylene glycol" which is another way of saying "poly-ethylene glycol" or PEG. [98]

27.4.2 Differential Diagnosis

Your doctor must rule out a diagnosis of constipation to eliminate the possibility of missing a serious condition than requires attention. These are the things to look for:

- Anal fissure
- Medication induced constipation
- Hypercalcemia
- Hypothyroidism
- Diabetes
- Spinal cord lesions
- Colonic strictures and blockages
- Colon cancer
- Parkinson disease

There are additional causes of constipation that are specific to children and infants, which are important to rule out with your pediatrician.

27.5 DIARRHEA ALTERNATING WITH CONSTIPATION

The symptoms of alternating constipation and diarrhea respond very well to GI Janel One.

The tricky part is the ramp up in dosing. If you start with a high dose or if you increase too quickly, you may cause some gassiness or cramping and think that it is not working. That is not the case. What is occurring is that you are increasing your dose too high or too quickly.

Remember that the digestive system is very delicate when you are having IBS/SIBO symptoms. It will respond to gentle support.

Since IBS/SIBO is multifactorial (meaning there can be many causes of the irritation), it is easy to see why many patients have a pattern that alternates constipation and diarrhea symptoms in addition to gassiness and abdominal pain.

You may have an underlying, ongoing irritation or deficit that causes constipation with episodes of exposure to something else (like a delayed food intolerance) that causes diarrhea. In these cases, there is often a good degree of retained stool in the bowels, as the bowel movements are so ineffective

GI irritation can be caused by a food, by a chronic undiagnosed infection in the small or large intestine, or both. It can also be a component when there is a deficiency or a structural deficit in the system.

To treat, start with your GI Janel Digest formulas

Step one:

- Take one or two capsules of GI Janel Digest A, B or C formula with each meal. Start with GI Janel Digest A. If tolerated, you can take up to six capsules of GI Janel Digest A with meals. If you experience any heartburn from taking one capsule of GI Janel Digest A, then stop and move to GI Janel Digest B. If you experience heartburn from this, then stop and move to GI Janel Digest C. If you know that you are sensitive, start with GI Janel Digest C.

Step two:

- Take one GI Jan-Aloe daily and as needed for pain or reflux

Step three:

- Use the soft food diet and Identify and remove food triggers (see the chapters on diet).

Step four:

- Add your GI Janel One gradually. See the GI Janel One dosing section for instructions. The special circumstance in this case is that you will only increase your GI Janel One to a maximum of three teaspoons (one tablespoon), unless you are treating gas and bloating in addition to alternating constipation/diarrhea. In that case, follow the standard GI Janel One dosing protocol.

- If your symptoms are *only* alternating diarrhea and constipation, and they persist after you achieve your three-teaspoon level of GI Janel One, then gradually add in acacia powder (see index for consultations with our doctors if required for your individual needs). Add in the acacia powder slowly in the same manner as the GI Janel One until you reach a dose of one heaping tablespoon twice daily. At this point you will be taking:

- GI Janel One: one tablespoon daily

- Acacia Fiber: Two tablespoons daily

- GI Janel Digest- A, B or C: with meals

- GI Jan-Aloe: One daily and one if needed for pain

GI Janel One contains the soluble fiber called acacia. Soluble fibers are very gentle and soothing to the digestive system. They are also prebiotics. Fiber feeds the beneficial bacteria that you want in your digestive system. These beneficial bacteria then take care of you!

If you have too little of these healthy bacteria or they are in the wrong place, and you add this fiber too quickly, the system can be overwhelmed, and you end up gassy and cramping. If you gradually increase your dose, you are coaxing the growth of the healthy bacteria and helping them to establish a strong ecosystem inside. The acacia is the most well-tolerated prebiotic and the only one I recommend for IBS/SIBO treatment. The other components of GI Janel One, help to strengthen your digestion so that any overgrowth of yeast and bacteria can simultaneously be balanced in the small and large intestine.

Soluble fibers turn to a gel-like substance in your body by absorbing water. This makes them soothing and protective to your system. The main fiber in GI Janel One is acacia fiber, which is derived from the gum of the Senegalia senegal tree

27.6. DIARRHEA

Here's a case of a 41-year-old health care worker who came in visibly distraught because, ever since having her gall bladder removed three years earlier, she would have instant and urgent diarrhea after eating. She told me that she had always had a sensitive digestive system and suffered from nausea as a child. She began to have episodes of digestive cramping pain two years after the removal of her gall bladder, but her gastroenterologist found nothing abnormal. Then she began to have upper digestive burning that was unresponsive to acid blockers. She said that her upper GI was bloated and burning (this is a classic SIBO hydrogen sulfide symptom).

At her first visit, she told me that food was pouring through her like water or pudding and she was having episodes of nausea with vomiting. She was already avoiding dairy and whole eggs as she had identified that these caused worsening of her diarrhea, bloating and pain. We decided to check for IgG food reactions in case there were more than dairy and egg causing problems. Meanwhile, I began her on GI Janel Digest B, GI Jan-Aloe for the upper GI burning, probiotics and activated charcoal. The previous GI work up did not include a test for inflammatory bowel disease, so we ran a fecal calprotectin to rule that out. This came back negative. I also asked her to use my soft food diet.

When she returned three weeks later, she told me that she started having regular bowel movements after one day of the supplements. Her bloating increased a little with the supplements at first, which I assured her was normal. The bloating and burning pain had since decreased. Her IgG results were positive for cow dairy and whole egg as she suspected. They were negative for gluten, but positive for wheat. They were highly positive for sugar, bakers' yeast and brewer's yeast. I asked her to eliminate and challenge these foods.

When I saw her again one month later, she had stopped her charcoal dosing, since it was causing constipation (for someone with a three-year history of urgent diarrhea, this can be a very welcome response). She had done a challenge with wheat and it did not cause symptoms. Otherwise she was not having any of the original symptoms. I began her on GI Janel One to strengthen and repair her digestive system so that symptoms would not return and requested that she gradually increase her dose to three teaspoons per day.

Three months later, she reported that she had no symptoms if she was using her GI Janel Digest B with meals and a maintenance dose of GI Janel One. She did add sugar and commercial baker's yeast intake to a couple of times a week without the return of symptoms. She did not want to add cow dairy or whole eggs back to her diet since the rest of her family avoided those anyway.

When considering the diarrhea and constipation of chronic IBS/SIBO conditions, the principles of both are not that different in terms of messages from your body. Bear with me here.

With functional constipation, your body is so irritated that peristaltic movement stops or is in a state of hyper spasm. The motion is ineffective to move the stool through the intestines. When your stools are narrow, it is due to the spasm and clenching of the colon. The functional constipation of IBS/SIBO is a sign of chronic irritation.

With diarrhea, your system is irritated when it encounters something it does not like and wants to get rid of it *fast*. In this case, the slow, steadiness of digestion is thrown off, and food moves through rapidly. This does not allow enough time for the breakdown of food or for water to be absorbed in the large intestine. The diarrhea of IBS/SIBO is a constant, acute irritation that has become long-term. Diarrhea can be very inefficient in its ability to clean out the bowels. Very often, a patient who has ongoing diarrhea will show signs of retained stool during abdominal exam, or abdominal imaging of their intestine will show pockets of retained stool.

Treatment of IBS/SIBO Diarrhea

Before embarking on your GI Janel journey, ensure that you have been properly tested for celiac disease, malabsorption, gastroenteritis, cancer and inflammatory bowel disease. These conditions are not the same as IBS/SIBO and require special treatment. People with inflammatory bowel disease should be treated by a gastroenterologist.

Step one:

- Take one or two capsules of GI Janel Digest A, B or C formula with each meal. Start with GI Janel Digest A. If tolerated, you can take up to six capsules of GI Janel Digest A with meals. If you experience any heartburn from taking one capsule of GI Janel Digest A, then stop and move to GI Janel Digest B. If you experience heartburn from this, then stop and move to GI Janel Digest C. If you know that you are sensitive, start with GI Janel Digest C.

Step two:

- Diet is critical for diarrhea: Use the soft food diet and eliminate all common food triggers. Especially important are dairy, gluten and whole eggs (see the chapter on diet).

Step three:

- Begin a high dose probiotic formula with the addition of Saccharomyces boulardii at the level of 5 billion CFU. Your total probiotic dose is between 100-200 billion organisms, 60 or more minutes between meals, in two divided doses. Your probiotic should not contain any FOS, fructo-oligosaccharides, inulin, sugars, or other added fibers.

Step four:

- Begin your GI Janel One dosing following the instructions in the dosing chapter. Stop at the level where your diarrhea resolves and hold it there.

Step five:

- If your symptoms do not gradually improve with the steps above, you will require functional stool testing (see the chapter on testing)

Step six:

- Once you have been diagnosed and treated for hidden, chronic infection, food intolerances or deficiencies based on the functional stool test results, if bloating and gassy symptoms remain, return to the GI Janel One treatment, which you will find in the dosing chapter for GI Janel One.

Here is a case of chronic diarrhea that responded very quickly to treatment. A 31-year-old woman, who had experienced a sensitive stomach and was prone to diarrhea her whole life, complained that her symptoms worsened at 18 when she started college. She had seen a gastroenterologist the year before her first visit with me, and both her endoscopy and colonoscopy were normal. She had reflux so badly that a temporary clip was placed in her esophagus to stop it. However she did not have obvious inflammation or gastritis on her scope. Her symptoms included severe diarrhea which continued even on three doses of Imodium per day. Immediately after food she would have cramping diarrhea, and saw the food she had just consumed in her stool. She had generalized abdominal pain that sometimes focused itself in the lower pelvic area. She had burning pain at her lower esophageal sphincter (reflux) and excessive gas that could become trapped and painful.

I immediately began her on GI Jan-Aloe daily and as needed for reflux symptoms. I began her on GI Janel One at ¼ teaspoon for seven days, and then ½ teaspoon per day while we waited for her IgG food test results. When I saw her four weeks later, she reported that her gas, reflux and diarrhea were all improving. She did have one episode of diarrhea after increasing her GI Janel One to the ½ teaspoon dose. I asked her to split her dose so that she took ¼ teaspoon twice daily or do a more gradual increase in dose. Her IgG results were positive for cow dairy, whole egg, sugar and gluten. She was also positive for almond, corn, peanut, and sesame, and had an overall pattern of leaky-gut syndrome. I did not ask her to remove foods from the second group. We discussed it, but she really did not want to give up the sugar, eggs, dairy or gluten from her diet, so we agreed to remove them for three months only and desensitize for foods so that she could resume eating them sooner.

When I saw her four weeks later, she told me that if she continues her supplements, regardless of what she eats, she does not have diarrhea, abdominal pain, reflux or gas. She did not need to remove dairy, gluten, sugar or eggs from her diet because the supplements alone were managing her symptoms well. We continued to desensitize her at eight-week intervals. During this time, she required a cholecystectomy to have her gall bladder removed. This made her more prone again to diarrhea when eating fat, so I added activated charcoal as a binder with higher fat meals. When I saw her after doing this, she told me that the charcoal was a miracle and she wished that she had known about it years ago. She said that it worked better for acute diarrhea than Imodium ever did.

My long-term goal, once we complete her desensitization, is to continue a maintenance dose of GI Janel One for the leaky gut repair and move her to GI Janel Digest B or C as her long-term treatment plan.

27.6.1 Differential Diagnosis

For acute diarrhea

27.6.1.1 *Viral*
Rotavirus, norovirus, enteric adenovirus, astrovirus

27.6.1.2 *Bacterial*
Campylobacter enteritis, shigella, salmonella, *Escherichia coli*, *Clostridium difficile*, *Yersinia*, *Vibrio cholerae*, *Staphylococcus aureus*, *Bacillus cereus*, *Clostridium perfringens*, listeria, *Aeromonas*, *Plesiomonas*, *Klebsiella oxytoca*.

27.6.1.3 *Parasitic*
Giardia, *Cryptosporidium*, *Microsporidiosis*, *Cyclospora*, *Isospora*

27.6.1.4 *Other causes*
Medications, radiation injury, malabsorption, ulcerative colitis, Crohn's disease, bowel ischemia.

For chronic diarrhea

27.6.1.5 *Colon-originated diarrhea*
- Ulcerative colitis, microscopic colitis (lymphocytic and collagenous), viral, bacterial and parasitic infections, HIV enteropathy, eosinophilic enteritis, chronic ischemic colitis, Infiltrating malignancy, graft versus host disease.

27.6.1.6 *Systemic causes*
- Drug side effects, alcohol, abetalipoproteinemia, advanced liver disease, common variable immune deficiency, amyloidosis

27.6.1.7 *Small-intestine origin*

- Celiac disease, Crohn's disease, bile salt malabsorption, brush border enzyme deficiency (lactose, fructose, sucrose, isomaltase), small intestinal bacterial overgrowth, radiation enteritis/colitis, NSAID enteropathy, protein losing enteropathy, Hodgkin lymphoma, Non-Hodgkin lymphoma, Tropical sprue, lymphangiectasia/impaired lymphatic drainage.

27.6.1.8 *Pancreatic*

- Pancreatic insufficiency

27.6.1.9 *Endocrine*

- Hyperthyroidism, diabetes mellitus, hypoparathyroidism, Addison disease, gastrinoma, carcinoid tumors, VIPoma.

27.6.1.10 *Other causes*

- Fecal impaction, surgical bypass or resection induced

28 Helpful tests

Many useful tests are now on the radar of functional and integrative doctors.

Many of these functional tests will be considered experimental by your insurance company and by conventional medicine. However, the tests I have included may be necessary to guide your treatment.

What I'm giving you here is my opinion after seeing thousands of GI patients, some of whom I've treated from the beginning of their diagnosis and some of whom have come in after years of symptoms with a stack of often-conflicting results from various labs.

Remember that there are three main issues we are dealing with when it comes to IBS/SIBO: food irritation, digestive deficiency, and hidden infection / microbiome balance and distribution.

I have designed my protocols to work without any testing, using your symptoms as a guide to a treatment that relieves, heals and replaces deficiency. Having said that, it is helpful and informative to determine if you have any unique food intolerances or hidden infections. If you decide to do some testing, the most important would be the IgG food antibodies by a specialty lab. These are now available as kits, which you can collect at home and then receive your results directly from the lab. I cannot recommend these at home kits at this point, until I have enough experience with these companies to determine their quality control.

28.1 IgG Antibody

For food reactions, I rely exclusively on IgG responses or in-office patch tests. For IBS/SIBO, all we need to know are reactions to dairy, whole eggs, sugar, yeast and gluten. Rarely, there are reactions to peanut, mushrooms, corn and soy. Occasionally the reaction will be to a specific gluten grain like wheat rather than spelt. High-starch carbohydrates may cause other carb intolerance symptoms, but rarely cause IgG antibody responses.

Since the IgG antibody panel is comprised of around 100 foods, some of the other foods which do not appear in the list above may be impacting other symptoms for you. But for the GI, you are looking for reaction from among the foods listed above. You will find a list of labs that perform this testing in the appendix which I have rated in terms of accuracy for detecting digestive problems.

As an example, I may get results back on a patient who is positive for IgG antibodies to dairy and whole eggs. When the GI Janel Digest formulas are used, and these foods are eliminated, much of the gas, diarrhea and bloating can be improved or resolved.

However, the same patient panel may be positive (and often is) for banana or cranberry. These may or may not be problems. These results are either false positives, cross reactions, or foods that are impacting other systems like the skin in terms of acne, rashes or eczema.

28.2 LEAKY GUT TESTS

Typically, I will use the IgG panel to determine the degree of leaky gut. This saves my patients from having to do a second test. An abundance of low-level reactions across the IgG panel indicates that most foods are interfacing with the immune system and triggering protective antibody expression. This has been a reliable method for determining foods to eliminate and the degree of permeability prior to the GI Janel protocol.

Other tests will check for zonulin and LPS (lipopolysaccharides) in the stool, which are markers for GI damage and inflammation. The reasoning behind this test is that zonulin is an integral part of the tight junctions and is a protein modulator of the gastrointestinal barrier. If found in excess in the stool sample, the junctions between the cells are in a state of damage and are releasing zonulin as a result. There are also blood tests for antibodies to zonulin. LPS are endotoxins from bacteria. It is reasoned that if these or antibodies to these can be found in testing, they are leaking in from the gut.

The older LGS tests are urine collections done after a challenge drink that tests for lactulose and mannitol transport through the GI wall. Mannitol is a small molecule and is easily absorbed through the gut wall in people with healthy intestinal linings. Lactulose is large and can be only minimally absorbed in a healthy system. A healthy intestinal lining will produce urine results with high mannitol and low lactulose recovery. Elevated levels of both in the urine indicates leaky gut. Low levels of both indicates malabsorption syndromes.

Following the GI Janel protocol, the zonulin or mannitol/lactulose challenge test is a good follow-up test after symptom resolution to determine whether you have completed the healing phase or longer treatment is required.

28.3 COMPREHENSIVE PARASITOLOGY STOOL TESTS

These tests (see Index) can be very helpful in the treatment of IBS-D or IBS- M / SIBO that is not responding well to the treatment protocols I have outlined in the treatment chapters. Insurance coverage varies and the labs that perform these tests are typically out of network. These are comprehensive tests and are unavailable through standard labs. They will measure, digestion and pancreatic output, nutrient absorption, inflammation and secretory IgA levels, microbiome distribution, overgrowth in terms of yeast, bacteria or parasites, and the desired bacterial levels of the colon.

28.4 IBSATUS TEST

This is a good bare-bones test for IBS. It will tell you if there are deficits in the digestive process, if there is active inflammation, or if there are any hidden infections and to what degree IgE food allergies are impacting digestion. It does not give any markers for IgG food intolerances and this would be the weakness of the test. It is essentially an abbreviated version of the comprehensive parasitology testing.

28.5 IBS DETEX

This is a relatively new test, which targets the post-infectious IBS symptoms. This test is an enzyme-linked immunosorbent assay (ELISA) that checks for antibodies that fight an acute infection.

These antibodies are cytolethal distending toxin B antibody and vinculin antibody. They are more commonly found in patients that have IBS-D (diarrhea) and IBS-M (mixed or alternating diarrhea / constipation)

This test is an attempt to have a definitive result indicating the diagnosis of IBS. These antibodies were found more commonly in patients with IBS-D relative to people with healthy digestion. Patients with other bowel diseases like IBD (inflammatory bowel disease) and some healthy patients were also found to have elevated levels of both these antibodies. Patients with celiac disease were found to commonly have elevated levels of cytolethal distending toxin B antibody. This test will not exclude a diagnosis of IBD (Crohn's disease or ulcerative colitis) and so it cannot be used to rule out this as a diagnosis.

28.6 BOWEL DISORDER EVALUATION RULE-OUT CASCADE

Some conventional labs offer a blood test that provides a panel to sequentially rule out Celiac disease, gluten sensitivity and inflammatory bowel disease. You may have more luck getting a test like this covered by your insurance and ordered by your MD if you are unable to work with a functional MD or ND. It would be a helpful place to start if your IBS/SIBO symptoms are primarily triggered by gluten intolerance.

28.7 SIBO TESTS

SIBO testing is not currently done by any in-network labs. The pricing varies depending on facility and the extent of the test offered. You will be required to follow dietary guidelines and preparation prior to the test. Then you will drink a challenge drink and collect breath samples for 2 or more hours. You will then send the breath samples into your lab for analysis. The test reveals the degree of gas (methane and hydrogen) produced when bacteria in the small intestine metabolize lactulose, fructose or glucose. The appearance of gas peaks during the sampling correspond to high areas of bacterial use of the sugar substrate.

Here's something interesting to consider. One of the leaky gut tests above uses absorption of lactulose (large molecule) as a test for permeability of the intestine. The more lactulose collected in the urine, the more is passing through the gastrointestinal barrier indicating intestinal inflammation damage or LGS. The same lactulose is used for SIBO testing. If you have both LGS and SIBO, will your SIBO test read low or false negative because the bacteria cannot ferment what is lost in absorption? Perhaps the next generation of SIBO testing will add urine lactulose collection with breath testing. We are also anticipating a SIBO test that adds in hydrogen sulfide as one of the measured gases.

28.8 LACTOSE INTOLERANCE BREATH TEST

This test will determine lactose intolerance. Remember that there are two main ways that an individual may adversely react to dairy when they are having ongoing GI symptoms. One is lactose intolerance (inability to breakdown the lactose sugar due to a deficit of lactase enzymes). The other is an inflammatory reaction to the protein in the dairy product which usually involves the IgG antibody pathways.

For the lactose breath test, a challenge drink of lactose is taken and then hydrogen and methane gases are collected for 3 or more hours. The higher the recovery of the gases, the greater the deficiency of lactase enzyme released in the small intestine. This causes symptoms of gas, bloating, diarrhea and abdominal pain when consuming lactose sugar in dairy products.

Lactose intolerance is most common in African, African American, Latino, Mediterranean, Jewish, Native American and Asian populations.

Lactose sugar is found in animal dairy products (cow, goat, and sheep). Lactose can break down in the fermentation process when making aged cheese (Cheddar, Parmesan, Swiss). Aged cheeses are better-tolerated due to their lower lactose content. Lactose is water soluble, so the higher the fat (like butter), the lower the lactose.

You may be both lactose-intolerant and diary protein-intolerant (casein, whey, lactalbumin). In this case, removing lactose alone will not stop you from reacting adversely to dairy.

28.9 STOOL YEAST TESTS

For patients who have constipation along with their gas and bloating or IBS-C / SIBO, a simple stool test from a conventional lab can determine if there is yeast overgrowth in the large intestine. Some of the labs will do a sensitivity test (to find out which anti-fungal will kill it). There are normal populations of yeast in the small and the large intestine. Unfortunately, there is currently no reliable method to determine small intestinal yeast overgrowth, apart from symptoms. However, as I've said earlier, those who have been positively diagnosed with SIBO have a high probability of also harboring SIFO (small intestinal yeast overgrowth) in the small intestine. Gassy symptoms can arise from the small intestine, large intestine, or both. Gassy symptoms can be due to SIBO, SIFO or both.

28.10 H PYLORI

Helicobacter pylori is the bacterial cause of gastrointestinal reflux and ulcers. H. pylori can easily be tested using a breath test or stool test and there are done by most conventional labs.

Historically, we would test the blood for the presence of *H. pylori* antibodies, but this test is not helpful since it does not differentiate whether the infection is current or past. Anyone who has either gastrointestinal reflux or ulceration of the stomach or small intestine should be tested for *H. pylori*.

28.11 COLONOSCOPY

A colonoscopy is performed as a procedure by a digestive specialist called a gastroenterologist. During this procedure, your doctor can determine if you have polyps growing, and then send them for a biopsy to see if they are benign, cancerous or have a high likelihood of becoming cancerous. This, along with your family history of colon cancer, will determine the frequency of your repeat colonoscopy procedures. The more likely you are to develop cancerous polyps, the more frequently you will need this procedure.

The colonoscopy will also check for inflammation, ulcerative colitis, Crohn's disease, eosinophilic disease, bleeding, granulomas, infections and adenomas. Sometimes problems with the appendix and problems with the ileocecal valve can be seen if the scope is able to advance that far. The colonoscopy will look at the colon which is the last three to five feet of the digestive system. The instrument is inserted into the rectum following sedation and a bowel cleanse. It is threaded along the colon and samples are collected as needed.

28.12 ENDOSCOPY EGD

An EGD is a procedure performed by your gastroenterologist. The endoscopy will look for celiac disease, inflammation, Crohn's disease, eosinophilic disease, bleeding, granulomas, infections and adenomas.

An EGD is a scope that enters through your mouth, and extends through the esophagus, stomach and into the first part of the small intestine. Samples are collected during the procedure and sent for biopsy to determine if there are any problems.

28.13 IMAGING OF THE SMALL INTESTINE

CT or MRI enterography is used to detect problems mainly for patients with Crohn's disease. MRI avoids the radiation risks of CT scan. This test can be ordered and performed at a diagnostic imagine facility.

28.14 OTHER DIAGNOSTIC IMAGING

CT of the abdomen and pelvis – A CT using contrast media can provide clinically useful information regarding ovarian pathology, pelvic inflammatory disease, ectopic pregnancy and ovarian torsion. It is indicated for lower left quadrant pain and suspected diverticular disease. It is indicated for diagnosing an abdominal mass, suspected appendicitis, liver metastases or suspected bowel obstruction.

Ultrasound of the abdomen – In pregnancy, this imaging is indicated for abdominal pain. A follow-up MRI can be done without contrast if the results are indeterminate. Abdominal ultrasound is also appropriate for jaundice with associated pain and fever. Abdominal ultrasound is used to check the pancreas and the gall bladder in the case of upper right quadrant pain and for examination of the pelvic reproductive system.

MRI – An abdominal MRI is used for liver follow-up when irregularities are found on ultrasound or CT scan. It is used in pregnancy and in children for right lower quadrant pain or suspected appendicitis.

MRI Fistulogram – Used for evaluation of perianal or perirectal fistulas.

Modified Barium Swallow – Used with dysphagia or difficulty swallowing.

29 CONVENTIONAL APPROACH TO IBS/SIBO

Your primary care provider (this may be an ND, MD, DO, NP or PA, depending on where you live) and gastroenterologist are important experts to help rule out serious digestive disorders that are life threatening. Your specialist may, depending on your symptoms and history, order some of the diagnostic testing above, do imaging or do a scope if indicated, either an EGD or a colonoscopy.

According to Epocrates, the definition of IBS is the condition of chronic abdominal pain with bowel dysfunction. The pain can be relieved by bowel movement and can be accompanied by abdominal bloating. There are no structural abnormalities. It occurs in about 15% of the adult population. It is further subdivided into IBS-D (diarrhea predominant), IBS-C (constipation predominant) or IBS-M (mixed).[99]

UpToDate medical resource defines SIBO as "a condition in which the small bowel is colonized by excessive aerobic and anaerobic microbes that are normally present in the colon. Most patients with SIBO present with bloating, flatulence, abdominal discomfort, or diarrhea.[100]

The conventional treatment plan for SIBO consists of antibiotics to reduce small intestinal bacteria. In addition, some patients require treatment of underlying nutritional deficiencies and associated ileitis/colitis.

Antibiotic therapy can be based on symptoms or testing. The selection of antibiotics is based on the pattern of bacterial overgrowth, the prevalence of risk factors for drug-resistance due to recent or repeated prior exposure, relevant antibiotic allergies, and cost. One of the main prescriptions used for SIBO is Xifaxan. The cost factor for the prescription of Xifaxan has been circumvented by the drug manufacturer offering discounts on treatment that substantially reduce the out of pocket cost to patients with insurance. The caveat for this benefit is that you must have a diagnosis of IBS-D. It is unnecessary to repeat breath testing if symptoms resolve with treatment.

In patients with hydrogen-predominant bacterial overgrowth without excess methane production, it is recommended to use rifaximin (Xifaxan) in divided doses of 1650 mg/day for 14 days. Rifaximin has a very low absorption into the body. It has been studied in effectiveness by the manufacturer to eliminate the symptoms of SIBO for up to six months. Repeated treatments are allowed for up to three times a year.

When I have done clinical cultures of colonic bacteria following the use of Xifaxan, in many cases I find an overgrowth of pathogens or potential pathogens. If the SIBO symptoms have improved, this indicates that there was an eradication of excessive bacterial species in the small intestine, an eradication of beneficial bacteria in the large intestine and a proliferation of unwanted bacterial species in the large intestine. I use this treatment with caution.

For patients with methane-predominant bacterial overgrowth, it is recommended to use a combination of neomycin 500 mg twice daily and rifaximin in divided doses of 1650 mg per day for 14 days.

There are simply not a lot of good answers for the symptoms of IBS/SIBO in conventional medicine with standard drug therapy. That is why so many people with these symptoms go for years with the abdominal symptoms and are asked to or decide to just live with them.

There are some medications that have been tried. However, these do not address the underlying functional issues and give minimal relief at best. Patients are often offered stress reduction techniques and are advised to eliminate coffee, lactose, sugar or fructose from their diets. The medications used in conventional medicine are generally symptomatic treatment. The drug treatment options are described in the following sections.

29.1 LAXATIVES

Rough, insoluble fiber laxatives, even those that are from a natural food source can be irritating to many IBS patients, especially early in treatment. These are commonly found in psyllium or flax fibers. Insoluble fiber can substantially increase gas and bloating.

MiraLAX is an *osmotic* laxative made of polyethylene glycol. It works by keeping more water in the colon. This makes the stools pass more easily when constipation is an issue. Polyethylene glycol is also a component in fuel and has other industrial uses. It has a low absorption into our blood stream when taken orally and has been approved by the FDA for use in adults and children over six months old for a period of two weeks or as directed by your doctor.

There are also formations of polyethylene glycol combined with electrolytes. These are often given for a bowel cleanse prior to colonoscopy.

Lactulose is an osmotic laxative. Do you recognize the name? It's the same substance used to test for SIBO and for gastrointestinal barrier damage or permeability.

Lubiprostone (Amitiza) and linaclotide (Linzess) are laxatives that work by increasing the movement of the intestine (motility) and the fluid secretion into the intestine.

Amitiza activates ClC-2 chloride channels, which increases intestinal fluid secretion and motility. This reduces intestinal permeability and stimulates recovery of mucosal barrier function.

Linzess activates the receptor guanylate cyclase-C, which stimulates cGMP production and increases intestinal fluid secretion and motility.

29.2 ANTI-SPASM MEDICATIONS

The anti-spasm drugs are in the chemical class called anti-cholinergic. This means they block the cholinergic response in the system, which decreases the spasm in the intestines. Anticholinergic drugs relax smooth muscle, decrease GI motility, and decrease gastric secretions.

The various generic drug names in this category are scopolamine, hyoscyamine, clidinium, atropine and dicyclomine. Dicyclomine also decreases bradykinin- and histamine-induced spasms. In some areas, anti-cholinergic drugs are combined with phenobarbital which is a barbiturate sedative. The brand Librax contains chlordiazepoxide which binds to benzodiazepine receptors and enhances GABA effects.

In my clinical experience, these medications can provide some symptom relief to patients. This can be helpful for a reprise in symptoms while we're uncovering the cause of the irritation and regenerating healthy intestinal function. Most of my patients stop their anti-spasm medications on their own, once their symptoms improve with the work we do together.

29.3 SELECTIVE SEROTONIN REUPTAKE INHIBITORS

Paroxetine (Paxil) and citalopram (Celexa) are in the family of medications that are prescribed for depression. They are in the family of SSRI or selective serotonin-reuptake inhibitor medications. These drugs decrease the breakdown of serotonin, keeping the levels of serotonin higher in the body. The theory behind this treatment rests on the prominent levels of serotonin located in the digestive system. I have seen these drugs be very helpful for mitigating the symptoms of depression, compulsion and anxiety, but they appear to have very limited benefit for gastrointestinal symptoms of IBS. Where they can help is by stabilizing the anxiety or obsessive compulsive (OCD) tendencies which may exacerbate the interpretation of IBS/SIBO symptoms and behavior.

29.4 TRICYCLIC ANTIDEPRESSANTS (TCA's)

Desipramine and amitriptyline inhibit norepinephrine and serotonin reuptake. Doxepin inhibits norepinephrine and serotonin reuptake. It also blocks central H1 receptors, so it makes you sleepier. The exact mechanism by which they relieve symptoms is unknown with these medications, but it is speculated to be an anticholinergic effect (see anti-spasm medications). They are used at lower doses for treating GI symptoms than when they are prescribed for depression. They can provide some symptom relief. The TCA's are dosed at bedtime due to their sedative effect. They can also cause constipation.

29.5 ANTI-DIARRHEA MEDICATION

Loperamide or Imodium works by binding to opioid receptors on the intestinal wall and inhibiting peristalsis (smooth muscle movement). It also increases anal sphincter tone. Imodium has been approved for acute or chronic (long term) use. It does, however carry a warning for the potential of paralysis of the intestines with long term use. This may lead to a condition called toxic mega colon or toxic colon. This is where there is stagnation and enlargement of the colon and a risk of perforation leading to sepsis. This is a medical emergency.[101]

Cholestyramine is an older drug that was originally used to lower cholesterol. It binds excess bile acids, so they do not irritate the intestine. It can be helpful in treating the cause of IBS-D if the patient has either an overproduction of bile acids or the inability to re-absorb bile acids. These bile acids in excessive amount irritate the intestine and cause diarrhea. Cholestyramine is also helpful in IBD or Inflammatory bowel disease (Crohn's disease and ulcerative colitis) when the intestines are inflamed and unable to re-absorb the bile acids. For IBD patients, this occurs due to tissue damage in the distal ileum (the final portion of the small intestine). It is helpful for diarrhea caused from the removal of the gall bladder and diarrhea caused by high fat diets.

29.6 SIBO Treatment

Xifaxan or Rifaximin is the current treatment for IBS-D.

Using an antibiotic to treat IBS-D was not a typical practice until the concept of the microbiome started gaining more attention. The first tests for SIBO (at the time called BOSI or Bacterial Overgrowth of the Small Intestine) came out in the 1990's and were available through one of the functional medical labs. Xifaxan was originally licensed by the FDA as a treatment for hepatic encephalopathy. Xifaxan is now approved for use in IBS-D by the FDA and is being widely marketed.

I personally reserve treatment of this severity for highly intractable patients. In the past years since its approval, I have prescribed it only a handful of times out of population base of thousands of IBS/SIBO patients. This is because it does not seem to resolve the problem permanently, and because I am concerned about killing off the entire microbiome to temporarily relieve symptoms. Studies done by the manufacturer of Xifaxan conclude that, symptoms can be relieved for up to six months. This was the length of their longest study period. The average relief from symptoms in clinical studies was ten weeks.

The Xifaxan manufacturer conducted double blind studies (meaning that both the patients and the providers did not know what was being given between the placebo and the treatment).

In the first study, the placebo group reported an improvement of abdominal pain and diarrhea of 39%. For the treatment group (Xifaxan) the improvement was 47%.

In the second study, the placebo group reported improvement of abdominal pain and diarrhea of 36% and the treatment group reported improvement of 47%. This is a statistically significant result and met with the criteria for FDA approval.[102]

The current protocol is to dose Xifaxan at 550 mg, three times a day for 14 days and when symptoms return, to repeat that protocol up to three times in a year. Previously the cost of this drug made this treatment prohibitive. However, since it's FDA approval for use in IBS-D this has become less of an issue. Use of

Xifaxan is an indication of how many patients are seeking answers that will help these chronic symptoms, even if that relief is temporary.

Xifaxan has not been approved as a treatment for SIBO. However, it is the main antibiotic treatment being prescribed at this time.

30 ADVANCED TREATMENT

For advanced treatment or questions, I recommend that you speak to one of our doctors on the GI Janel Team. Some patients will require additional diagnostics or advanced treatment in terms of natural or prescription therapy, which is beyond the scope of this book.

We offer remote visits to answer questions and personalize your treatment experience. Information on this can be found on the GI Janel Anywhere website (https://consult.gijanel.com/). Telemedicine visits allow us to personalize your treatment plan and recommend further supplement intervention through our online pharmacy. Our doctors support dietary questions and will coach you in the nuances of your personal treatment successes.

If appropriate, immunotherapy may be recommended as an in-office treatment. At this time, we have many patients who travel for their immunotherapy every two months, so they may more successfully add foods back to their diet.

31 APPENDIX

31.1 LABORATORIES IgG TESTING:

US BioTek Laboratories, Inc. (https://usbiotek.com)

Meridian Valley Lab (https://www.meridianvalleylab.com) (less accurate)

31.2 LABORATORIES STOOL TESTING:

LabCorp (https://www.labcorp.com)

Quest Diagnostics (https://questdiagnostics.com)

Genova Diagnostics (https://www.gdx.net)

Diagnostic Solutions Laboratory GI Map (https://www.diagnosticsolutionslab.com/tests/gi-map)

The Great Plains Laboratory, Inc. (https://www.greatplainslaboratory.com)

Doctor's Data, Inc. (https://www.doctorsdata.com)

DiagnosTechs (https://www.diagnostechs.com)

31.3 LABORATORIES SIBO TESTING

Genova Diagnostics (https://www.gdx.net)

SIBOTest (https://sibotest.com)

Many are available with an online search and do not require a doctor's order

31.4 Labs- H pylori Testing

LabCorp (https://www.labcorp.com)

Quest Diagnostics (https://questdiagnostics.com)

Genova Diagnostics (https://www.gdx.net)

31.5 Lactose Intolerance Testing

LabCorp (https://www.labcorp.com)

Quest Diagnostics (https://questdiagnostics.com)

Genova Diagnostics (https://www.gdx.net)

31.6 IBS Detex

True Health Labs (https://www.truehealthlabs.com)

Quest Diagnostics (https://questdiagnostics.com)

31.7 LGS Test

Cyrex Zonulin (https://www.cyrexlabs.com)

Cyrex Intestinal permeability panel including LPS levels (https://www.cyrexlabs.com)

31.8 ORGANIC ACID TEST

The Great Plains Laboratory, Inc.
(https://www.greatplainslaboratory.com)

Genova Diagnostics (https://www.gdx.net)

31.9 MYCOTOXIN TESTS

The Great Plains Laboratory, Inc.
(https://www.greatplainslaboratory.com)

31.10 SHOPPING LIST

Vegetables – carrots, yams, sweet potato, potato, spinach, avocado, asparagus, artichoke, green beans, beets, parsnip, turnip, Swiss chard.

Proteins – turkey, chicken, fish, beef, buffalo, bison, lamb, protein powders (rice or hemp), protein bars (low sugar, low fiber), bones for bone broth, hemp hearts.

Soft fruits – berries, bananas, plums, peaches, apricots, avocado, mango, papaya, ripe melon

Hard fruits for sauces or baking – Apples, Pears

Nut and Seed Butters – hazelnut, cashew, tahini (sesame), walnut, almond, pine, Brazil, sunflower, pumpkin, pistachio, mixed nuts and seeds. You can make your own nut or seed butter from the whole nuts. To do this, blend nuts in a processor until smooth. You could also add water to make nut milk, or add a sweetener, then freeze the nut milk to make nut ice cream.

Condiments – sea salt or other whole salt, earth balance original tub (earthbalancenatural.com), dairy free, soy free spread, Daiya dairy free cream cheese or other Cheese and Milk free products (daiya.com), mustard, horseradish, fresh herbs, tamari or soy sauce, Bragg Liquid Aminos, any gluten and dairy free dressing or egg-free condiment like Veganaise (followyourheartproducts.com), avocado mayonnaise, nut or seed butters.

Cold Pressed Oils – olive, almond, sesame, sunflower, avocado, safflower, coconut, grapeseed. Avoid chemically extracted or heat-extracted oils. Use polyunsaturated oils cold (Olive) and monounsaturated (Avocado, Ghee) for heating on high heat.

Online shopping:

Thrivemarket.com – all types of food available

Brandless.com – all types of food available

Earthbalancenatural.com – spreads, butters, dressings, snacks

Daiya.com – cheese, yogurts, dressing, sauces

Followyourheartproducts.com – mayonnaise substitutes, dips, spreads, sauces, vegan cheese

KiteHill.com (DF)

Glutino.com (GF)

Schaer.com (GF)

BFree (GF ciabatta)

AllergyFreeMenuPlanners.com

EatingWithFoodAllergies.com

ShopWell Diet scanner (app)

Online searches for dairy free, gluten-free foods and apps

31.10.1 Adding grain carbohydrates:

White rice: basmati

Quinoa

Oats

Teff pancakes (Ethiopian)

Cassava tortillas

Rice or quinoa pastas, crackers

Small batch sour dough bread

31.10.2 Adding gluten-free breads:

Breads, buns, rolls, biscuits, cereals, pancakes, waffles, soft crackers, tortillas, wraps. Use products with a simple and short ingredient list. Limit complex ingredients in gluten free products as the gums and emulsifiers can result in diarrhea and abdominal pain for those with sensitive digestion. Small batch (local bakery) sourdough can be tolerated very well, even by those who cannot tolerate gluten.

Dairy, egg, gluten, soy, corn, yeast: Use these only if you have tested IgG negative by a reliable lab and you know you don't react to them or have challenged them for reaction.

31.11 AVOID THE DIRTY DOZEN:

Buying organic is always the best. It is also good to buy locally farmed food or at the very minimum stateside farmed produce. The following is the EWG.org (Environmental Working Group) Dirty Dozen guide to items that should always be purchased organic if possible, to avoid the pesticide residue.

Strawberries	Cherries
Spinach	Peaches
Nectarines	Pears
Apples	Grapes
Tomatoes	Celery
Potatoes	Sweet bell peppers

31.12 MEAL ASSEMBLY

Have you ever noticed that when you eat at restaurant from a certain culture, the options are combinations of very similar ingredients that are combined in different ways? A Vietnamese salad roll and a Vietnamese noodle salad are the same ingredients, arranged differently. An enchilada and a taco are a different preparation of the same ingredients. Following this same principle, listed below are options that can turn your limited food list into unique meals that you can eat at the table or on the go.

Bowls

1. White rice or quinoa or mashed potato as base

2. Add well-cooked or pureed veggies

3. Add protein

4. Top with your condiment

For example:

1. Quinoa

2. Cooked Spinach

3. Grilled salmon w/ lemon and sea salt

Soups:

1. Chicken or veggie or bone broth

2. Add white rice or quinoa

3. Add cooked veggies

4. Add chopped protein

For example:

1. Chicken broth

2. Cooked White Rice

3. Cooked carrots

4. Diced roasted chicken breast

Wraps

1. Rice wrap, Corn Tortilla, Gluten Free wrap or butter lettuce leaves

2. Add protein

3. Add Soft Veggies

4. Add healthy fat – chopped nuts, avocado

5. Add condiment or nut butter

For example:

1. Rice, Teff or Cassava wrap

2. Turkey slices

3. Arugula, basil and Heirloom tomato

4. Sliced avocado

5. Veganaise Dressing.

Plates

1. Protein

2. Starch: sweet potato, white rice or quinoa

3. Well-cooked veggies

4. Healthy fat (fish, olive oil, avocado, nuts butter)

For example:

1. Grass fed beef

2. Sweet potato mashed with dairy free spread and sea salt

3. Asparagus, well sautéed with olive oil, garlic and sea salt

Salads

1. Soft leafy greens

2. Add soft chopped/julienned veggies

3. Add protein

4. Dress and season – lemon or lime juice and extra virgin olive oil, herbs if desired: oregano, basil, dill, mint

For example:

1. Baby arugula, baby spinach, butter lettuce

2. Well-cooked and chilled beets, carrots and asparagus

3. Diced chicken

4. Dress with Lemon, olive oil and basil

Shakes

Blend:

- Rice or hemp-based, bone broth based or Essential Amino Acid Protein Powder
- ½ cup frozen, organic berries or other soft fruit
- 1 cup coconut milk or another dairy alternative
- ½ cup ice

Add-ins:

- Nut or seed butter
- Avocado
- Coconut cream (canned)

Snacks

- Apple or pear sauce
- Nut or seed butter with Rice
- Soft cracker or bread with hummus/vegan cheese/soft fruit
- Turkey avocado roll up
- Shakes
- Low-fiber and low-sugar protein bar
- Rice/quinoa cakes with tree nut butter or fruit
- Dairy free pudding, ice creams or yogurt

31.13 PROBIOTICS

Pur-Biome (Pure Encapsulations) diarrhea specific

Therbioitic (Klaire brand)

Othobiotic (Orthomolecular products)

Flora 200-14 and 20-14 (Innate brand)

31.14 SUPPLEMENTS THAT CAN IRRITATE IBS/SIBO

While the theory behind the use of some of the following is reasonable and compelling, I have seen the following list of supplements do absolutely nothing for symptoms at best and irritate or increase symptoms at worst.

Mastic Gum

While this may be helpful for isolated cases of Reflux Disease and Gastric or Duodenal Ulceration, it can be very irritating and painful in some cases for IBS/SIBO patients.

FOS (fructo oligo saccharides, galactooligosaccharides)

There are now many probiotics produced without prebiotics like FOS. These are a better choice due to the easy fermentation and gas produced with oral intake of FOS.

Other Prebiotics

Other fibers like resistant starch, pectin, beta glycan and xylooligosaccharies are often easily fermented and can increase the symptoms of gas and bloating. They are not helpful to use until the main symptoms of gas and bloating have been resolved. They can then be added in slowly and gradually to promote the growth of desired bacterial species.

Glutamine

Glutamine can increase diarrhea and loosen stools. It is considered the main protein nutrient in theory, but in practice does little to resolve symptoms. I would use it only after gas, bloating, diarrhea and pain are resolved to potentially maintain cellular health.

Butyrate

This stuff smells awful. If it even makes it all the way through to the large intestine, I have seen it do very little to improve symptoms.

31.15 THERAPEUTIC CASTOR OIL PACK

This is a soothing treatment to aid in the gentle relief of abdominal pain, stagnation and constipation.

REQUIRED ITEMS

1.   Pure, cold-pressed castor oil (not chemically or heat extracted)

2.   Towel/facecloth to cover size of the area (when folded in double thickness)

3.   Heating pad

4.   Plastic wrap

Directions:

1.   Soak Towel in castor oil and heat in microwave or oven and place on the entire abdomen. Check that the temperature is not too hot before placing on your body.

2.   Place plastic over pack (to prevent staining of linens and clothing) and cover with heating pad.

3.   Cover with a dry towel or something to hold pack in place if needed

5.   Leave pack in place for between one hour or longer (the longer the better).

6.   While treatment is being applied, rest comfortably or sleep.

        Store pack in a zip-lock bag in the refrigerator or cupboard if using daily. It may be reused 30 times by adding oil to keep saturated.

Frequency: One hour or longer (The longer the better. You can wear it to bed)

Abdominal Benefits

Therapeutic oils have been used for centuries to relieve pain and regenerate the body. These oils can penetrate the skin layers, entering the lymphatic channels (waste cleaning system), which surround the abdominal organs. Here the oils promote an increase in the activity and quantity of white blood cells (the immune protective cells). The lymphatics are then more enabled to shunt chemical stagnation out of the area. They additionally act as an anti-inflammatory, reducing chemical pain messengers, soothing damage and promoting deep healing. When applied to the liver, there is an increase in activity of detoxification biochemistry and liver regeneration. This is a lipoatrophic effect, promoting the liver to remove toxins from your body.

Injuries or Pain

As castor oil is absorbed through the skin, it moves through the lymphatic channels, allowing the breakup of congestion. Since the pain and swelling from injury is due, in great part to the interruption of lymph drainage in the affected area, resulting in an accumulation of fluid, this action on the lymphatics makes this oil a valuable first aid tool and sinus treatment.

31.16 FOOD IMMUNOTHERAPY

My preferred protocol is to use in office immunotherapy treatments to resolve food intolerance. I treat patients for six to twenty-four visits, and then have my patients begin to use food at home to continue the building of their tolerance and re-introduction of a food type. This immunotherapy increases the T regulator cell population to foods so there is a decreased inflammatory response. Introducing small amounts of the offending foods following this treatment, continues the generation of the T regulator cell population.

At-home food immunotherapy is then continued by having tiny amounts of the intolerant food (1teaspoon to 1 tablespoon) on a weekly basis and gradually adding in regular servings as frequently as tolerated. Your body tells you if it's had too much of a food or if it's not ready for it at all. Seeing small amounts of the food can continue to teach the body to increase the T regulatory cell population.

More can be found about in-office immunotherapy to food reactions on my website specialtynaturalmedicine.com.

31.17 FOOD CHALLENGE

The food challenge is simply done by removing a food or group of foods for two weeks, then consuming large amounts of that food type for one day and then waiting for five days to track any delayed reactions.

Immediate reactions are obvious. When I get IgG panels back from patients and they are reactive to more than one food, we use this method to determine which are the actual food issues and which are secondary reactions or false positive reactions and do not need to be avoided. This simplifies the dietary restrictions for GI healing and makes life much less complicated as we employ the GI Janel formulas to promote equilibrium, symptom relief and homeostasis.

32 REFERENCES

1 (Afshar-Sterle, 2014)
2 (Rao, 2018)
3 (Bowen, 2016)
4 (Bowen, 2015)
5 (Journal, 2011)
6 (Christoph A. Thaiss, 2016, July)
7 (Bowen, 2016)
8 (Anon., 2016)
9 (Gillman, 2016)
10 (Anon., 2018)
11 (King, 2009)
12 (Berger & Gray, 2009)
13 (Holzer, 2007)
14 (Biancani, 2006)
15 (Fisher & Cohen, 1973)
16 (MacKay Douglas & Miller, 2003)
17 (Stiefel & Donskey, 2006)
18 (Delaney & Suissa, 2005)
19 (Laheij, 2004)
20 (Yang X & D.C, 2006)
21 (JM, et al., 2004)
22 (Bowen, 2014)
23 (Bowen, n.d.)
24 (US National Library of Medicine, 2018)
25 (Evans, et al., 1988)
26 (Gov, 2011)
27 (Organs of the Body, 2018)
28 (Feltman, 2014)
29 (Diagnostic Solutions, 2018)
30 (Anon., 2018)
31 (Epocrates, 2018)
32 (Ford, et al., 2014)
33 (Kuhnlein, 2009)
34 (Guardian , 2014)
35 (Slazenger, 2015)
36 (Hebbar, 2018)
37 (Gominak, 2017)
38 (American Society for Microbiology, 2008)
39 (Night, 2017)
40 (Carnahan, 2018)
41 (Gominak, 2017)
42 (WebMD, 2018)
43 (Sutter Health, 2012)
44 (Nigh, 2017)
45 (Cohen, et al., 1973)
46 (Donohue, 2010)
47 (Dharmananda, 2005)
48 (Dharmananda, 2005)

[49] (Web MD, 2018)
[50] (Australian Society of Clinical Immunolgy and Allergy , 2014)
[51] (Gerhardt, 2006)
[52] (Wikibooks, 2014)
[53] (Jacob, 2003)
[54] (University of Chicago , 2018)
[55] (Conde Naste, 2014)
[56] (Terzcak, 2013)
[57] (Grainstorm , 2018)
[58] (Anderson, 2018)
[59] (Hoffenberg, 2018)
[60] (Thermo Scientific, 2012)
[61] (Fiocchi & Fierro, 2017)
[62] (Fedewa & Rao, January 2014)
[63] (Quizlet, 2018)
[64] (Raszkowski, et al., 1976)
[65] (Iozzo & Schaefer, 2015)
[66] (Ophardt, 2003)
[67] (Brown & Klauder, Arch Derm Syphilol. 1933;27(4):584-604)
[68] (University of Leeds, 2015)
[69] (Millipore Sigma, 2018)
[70] (Bowen, 2018)
[71] (Titanbiotech , 2018)
[72] (Bilal, 2008)
[73] (Wolters Kluwer Health, 2009)
[74] (Spencer, 2014)
[75] (Singh & Lin, 2015)
[76] (Weld & Gunther, 1947)
[77] (Cooper & Williams, 2004, August)
[78] (Chemeurope, 2018)
[79] (Seneff, 2011)
[80] (Sisson, 2012)
[81] (Silver Colloids, 2012)
[82] (Seneff, 2011)
[83] (Noker, et al., 2001)
[84] (Cornell, 1995)
[85] (Seneff, 2017)
[86] (MSM Epocrates, 2018)
[87] (Lee, 1999)
[88] (Otten, et al., 2006)
[89] (Lee, 2008)
[90] (Clarke & Sperandio, June 1, 2005)
[91] (Dockrill, 2008)
[92] (Stiefel & Donskey, 2006)
[93] (Delaney & Suissa, 2005)
[94] (Laheij, 2004)
[95] (Yang X & D.C, 2006)
[96] (Ruskin & Vakuck, 2012 May)
[97] (Vakuck & Ruskin, 2004 April)
[98] (Center for Disease Control, 2011)
[99] (Epocrates, 2018)
[100] (Pimentel, 2018)
[101] (Lin & Cagir, 2018)

[102] (Saadi & McCallum, 2013)

BIBLIOGRAPHY

Afshar-Sterle, D. Z. N. J. B. A. K. S. L. R. e. a., 2014. *Fas ligand-medicated immune survelliance by T cells is essential for the control of spontaneous B cell lymphomas.* s.l., s.n., p. DOI: 10.1038/nm.3442.

American Society for Microbiology, 2008. *Humans Have Ten Times More Bacteria Than Human Cells: How Do Microbial Communities Affect Human Health?.* [Online]
Available at: https://www.sciencedaily.com/releases/2008/06/080603085914.htm

Anderson, J., 2018. *Is Sourdough gluten free.* [Online]
Available at: https://www.verywellfit.com/is-sourdough-bread-gluten-free-562853

Anon., 2016. *Cell Biology at Yale.* [Online]
Available at: http://medcell.med.yale.edu/lectures/epithelial_structure.php

Anon., 2016. *Cell Biology at Yale.* [Online]
Available at: http://medcell.med.yale.edu/lectures/epithelial_structure.php

Anon., 2018. *Cell Biology Introduction.* [Online]
Available at: https://en.wikibooks.org/wiki/Cell_Biology/Introduction/Cell_size

Anon., 2018. *Small Intestine.* [Online]
Available at: https://microbewiki.kenyon.edu/index.php/Small_Intestine

Australian Society of Clinical Immunolgy and Allergy , 2014. *Sulfite Sensitivity.* [Online]
Available at: https://allergy.org.au/patients/product-allergy/sulfite-allergy

Berger, M. & Gray, J. R. B., 2009. *The expanded biology of seratonin, Annual review of medicine.* [Online]
Available at: https://www.ncbi.nlm.nih.gov/pubmed/19630576

Biancani, P. P. H. K. M. P., 2006. *GI Motility online.* [Online]
Available at: https://www.nature.com/gimo/contents/pt1/full/gimo24.html

Bilal, A., 2008. *The role of copper- and sulfur- based fungicides in organic vegetable production.* [Online]
Available at: http://www.farmstart.ca/wp-content/uploads/2008/05/ahmed-article-inorganic-fungicides-04-25-2008.pdf

Bowen, R., 2014. *Absorption of Lipids.* [Online]
Available at:

http://www.vivo.colostate.edu/hbooks/pathphys/digestion/smallgut/absorb_lipids.html

Bowen, R., 2015. *Absorption of minerals and metals.* [Online]
Available at:
http://www.vivo.colostate.edu/hbooks/pathphys/digestion/smallgut/absorb_minerals.html

Bowen, R., 2016. *Absorption of Monosaccharides.* [Online]
Available at:
http://www.vivo.colostate.edu/hbooks/pathphys/digestion/smallgut/absorb_sugars.html

Bowen, R., 2016. *The Gastrointestinal Barrier.* [Online]
Available at:
http://www.vivo.colostate.edu/hbooks/pathphys/digestion/stomach/gibarrier.html

Bowen, R., 2018. *GI Barrier.* [Online]
Available at:
http://www.vivo.colostate.edu/hbooks/pathphys/digestion/stomach/gibarrier.html

Bowen, R., n.d. *Fermentation Chemistry.* [Online]
Available at:
http://www.vivo.colostate.edu/hbooks/pathphys/digestion/herbivores/ferment.html

Brown, H. B. & Klauder, J. V., Arch Derm Syphilol. 1933;27(4):584-604. *SULPHUR CONTENT OF HAIR AND OF NAILS IN ABNORMAL STATES.* [Online]
Available at: https://jamanetwork.com/journals/jamadermatology/article-abstract/510932

Carnahan, J. N., 2018. *6 signs that SIBO may be the root cause of your IBS.* [Online]
Available at: https://www.jillcarnahan.com/2014/05/16/6-signs-sibo-might-root-cause-ibs/

Center for Disease Control, 2011. *Ethylene Glycol.* [Online]
Available at:
https://www.cdc.gov/niosh/ershdb/EmergencyResponseCard_29750031.html

Chemeurope, 2018. *Disulfide Bonds.* [Online]
Available at:
http://www.chemeurope.com/en/encyclopedia/Disulfide_bond.html

Christoph A. Thaiss, N. Z., 2016, July . The microbiome and innate immuntiy.. *Nature, International Journal of Science* , p. https://www.nature.com/articles/nature18847.

Christoph A. Thaiss, N. Z. M. L. &. E. E., 2016. *The microbiome and innate immunity.* [Online]
Available at: https://www.nature.com/articles/nature18847

Clarke, M. B. & Sperandio, V., June 1, 2005. Events at the Host-Microbial Interface of the Gastrointestinal Tract III. Cell-to-cell signaling among microbial flora, host, and pathogens: there is a whole lot of talking going on. *American Journal of Physiology Gastrointestinal and Liver Physiology,* p. 288: G1105–G1109.

Cohen, H. J., Drew, R. T., Johnson, J. L. & Rajagopalan, K. V., 1973. *Molecular Basis of the Biological Function of Molybdenum. The Relationship between Sulfite Oxidase and the Acute Toxicity of Bisulfite and SO2.".* s.l., Bibcode:1973PNAS...70.3655C. PMC 427300 . PMID 4519654. doi:10.1073/pnas.70.12.3655 , p. 70 (12 Pt 1–2): 3655–3659.

Conde Naste, 2014. *cereals grains and pastas.* [Online]
Available at: https://nutritiondata.self.com/facts/cereal-grains-and-pasta/9265/2

Cooper, R. & Williams, J., 2004, August. Elemental sulphur as an induced antifungal substance in plant defence.. *Journal of Experimental Botany* , pp. 55(404):1947-53.

Cornell, 1995. *Sulfur.* [Online]
Available at: http://pmep.cce.cornell.edu/profiles/extoxnet/pyrethrins-ziram/sulfur-ext.html

Delaney, S. D. & Suissa, B. A., 2005. Use of gastric acid suppressive agents and the risk of community aquired Clostridium difficle-associated disease. *JAMA,* pp. Dec 21; 294(23):2989-95.

Dharmananda, S. P., 2005. *Differentiating Sulfur Compounds Sulfa Drugs, Glucosamine Sulfate, Sulfur, and Sulfiting Agents.* [Online]
Available at: http://www.itmonline.org/arts/sulfa.htm

Diagnostic Solutions, 2018. *Interpretive Guide.* [Online]
Available at: diagnosticsolutionslab.com

Dockrill, P., 2008. *Acid relux drug proton pum inhibitors medication risk of stoamch cancer.* [Online]
Available at: https://www.sciencealert.com/acid-reflux-drug-proton-pump-inhibitors-medication-risk-stomach-cancer-helicobacter

Donohue, M. J., 2010. *The Detoxification System Part III: Sulfoxidation and Sulfation.* [Online]

Available at: http://www.talkingaboutthescience.com/studies/Donohue-Sulfoxidation.pdf

Epocrates, 2018. *IBS*. [Online]
Available at: https://online.epocrates.com/diseases/12221/Irritable-bowel-syndrome/Definition

Evans, D. et al., 1988. *Measurement of gastrointestinal pH profiles in normal ambulant human subjects..* [Online]
Available at: https://www.ncbi.nlm.nih.gov/pmc/articles/PMC1433896/

Fedewa, A. & Rao, S. S., January 2014. Dietary fructose intolerance, fructan intolerance and FODMAPs. *Current Gastroenterology Reports* , p. 16(1): 370..

Feltman, R., 2014. *The Gut's Microbiome Changes Rapidly with Diet.* [Online]
Available at: https://www.scientificamerican.com/article/the-guts-microbiome-changes-diet/

Fiocchi, A. M. & Fierro, V. M., 2017. *Food Allergy.* [Online]
Available at: http://www.worldallergy.org/education-and-programs/education/allergic-disease-resource-center/professionals/food-allergy

Fisher, R. M. & Cohen, S. M., 1973. *Physiological Characteristics of the Human Pyloric Sphincter.* [Online]
Available at: https://www.gastrojournal.org/article/S0016-5085(73)80092-7/abstract

Ford, A. C. M. C. M. F. 1., Moayyedi, P. B. M. C. P. M. F. 2. & Lacy, B. E. ,. M. P., 2014. *American College of Gastroenterology Monograph on the Management of Irritable Bowel Syndrome and Chronic Idiopathic Constipation.* [Online]
Available at: http://gi.org/wp-content/uploads/2014/08/IBS_CIC_Monograph_AJG_Aug_2014.pdf

Gerhardt, A. M., 2006. *SULFA, SULFITE, SULF-WHATEVER ALLERGIES.* [Online]
Available at:
http://www.healthychoicesformindandbody.org/Medisense_Articles/06096-Sulfa_Allergy.pdf

Gillman, C., 2016. *FDA Tests Confirm Oatmeal, Baby Foods Contain Residues of Monsanto Weed Killer.* [Online]
Available at: https://www.huffingtonpost.com/carey-gillam/fda-tests-confirm-oatmeal_b_12252824.html

Gominak, S. M., 2017. *Vitamin D Sleep Gut Bacteria and Methylation* [Interview] 2017.

Gov, N. Z., 2011. *Large Intestine Function*. [Online]
Available at: https://www.sciencelearn.org.nz/resources/1832-large-intestine-function

Grainstorm , 2018. *baking mixes*. [Online]
Available at: https://grainstorm.com/collections/baking-mixes

Guardian , 2014. *Indigenous diets fight modern illnesses*. [Online]
Available at: https://www.theguardian.com/global-development/2014/feb/03/indigenous-diets-fight-modern-illnesses

Hebbar, D. J., 2018. *Castor Oil Benefit and use research*. [Online]
Available at: https://easyayurveda.com/2014/12/12/castor-benefits-use-research-side-effects/

Hoffenberg, E. J. M., 2018. *Celiac Disease in Children*. [Online]
Available at: https://celiac.org/about-celiac-disease/celiac-disease-in-children/

Holzer, P., 2007. Taste Receptors in the Gastrointestinal Tract. V. Acid sensing in the gastrointestinal tract. *Gastrointestinal and Liver Physiology*, pp. G669-G705.

Holzer, P., 2007. Taste Receptors in the Gastrointestinal Tract. V. Acid sensing in the gastrointestinal tract. *Gastrointestinal and Liver Physiology* , pp. G669-G705.

Iozzo, R. V. & Schaefer, L., 2015. *Proteoglycan form and function: A comprehensive nomenclature of proteoglycans, Matrix Biology*. [Online]
Available at:
https://www.sciencedirect.com/science/article/pii/S0945053X15000402

Jacob, S. W. M. F., 2003. *MSM-The Definitive Guide - A Comprehensive Review of the Science and Therapeutics of Methylsulfonylmethan* [Interview] 2003.

JM, R., 2nd, P. R. & RJ., V., 2004. Vitamin B12 deficiency associated with histamine (2) receptor antagonists and proton-pump inhibitor. *Journal of Clinical Epidemiology* , p. Apr; 57(4):4.

Journal, A. J. C. B., 2011. *Intestinal Absorption of water-soluble vitamins in health and disease*. [Online]
Available at: http://www.biochemj.org/content/437/3/357

King, M., 2009. *An Overview of the human nervous system*. [Online]
Available at: http://themedicalbiochemistrypage.org/nerves.html

Kuhnlein, H., 2009. *Indigenous Nutrition*. [Online]
Available at: http://indigenousnutrition.org/

Laheij, R. e. a., 2004. Risk of community acquired pneumonia and use of gastric acid-suppressive drugs.. *JAMA*, pp. Oct 27: 1955-1060.

Lee, M., 2008. *Major Sources of Dietary Sulfur.* [Online]
Available at: https://healthyeating.sfgate.com/major-sources-dietary-sulfur-4924.html

Lee, T. S., 1999. *Cellular Matrix Study.* [Online]
Available at: http://www.naturodoc.com/sulfurstudy.htm

Lin, B. & Cagir, B. M. F., 2018. *Toxic Megacolon.* [Online]
Available at: https://emedicine.medscape.com/article/181054-overview

MacKay Douglas, N. & Miller, A. L. N., 2003. *Nutritional support for wound healing, Alternative Medicine Review.* [Online]
Available at:
https://www.spectracell.com/media/uploaded/0/0e2034897_011fullpaper2003alt medrevnutritionalsupportforwoundhealingpdfpdf-.pdf

Millipore Sigma, 2018. *Glycosaminoglycans and proteoglycans.* [Online]
Available at: https://www.sigmaaldrich.com/technical-documents/articles/biology/glycobiology/glycosaminoglycans-and-proteoglycans.html

MSM Epocrates, 2018. *Methylsulfonylmethane Monograph.* [Online]
Available at: https://online.epocrates.com/drugs/alternative-medicines/717208/methylsulfonylmethane/Monograph

Nigh, G. N., 2017. *SIBO and hydrogen sulfide* [Interview] (20 December 2017).

Noker, K. et al., 2001. Toxicity of Methylsulfonylmethane in rats. *Food Chemical Toxicology*, pp. 40: 1459-1462.

Ophardt, C. E., 2003. *Quaternary Protein Structure, Virtual Chem Book.* [Online]
Available at: http://chemistry.elmhurst.edu/vchembook/567quatprotein.html

Organs of the Body, 2018. *Large Intestine Function in Human Digestive System.* [Online]
Available at: http://www.organsofthebody.com/large-intestine/large-intestine-function.php

Otten, J. J., Pitzi Hellwig, J. & Meyers, L. D., 2006. *Dietary Reference Intakes: The Essential Guide to Nutrient Requirements..* Washington DC: The National Academies Press..

Pimentel, M. M. F., 2018. *small intestinal bacterial overgrowth management.* [Online]
Available at: https://www.uptodate.com/contents/small-intestinal-bacterial-

overgrowth-
management?source=search_result&search=sibo&selectedTitle=1~136

Quizlet, 2018. *Connective Tissue.* [Online]
Available at: https://quizlet.com/184698393/connective-tissue-flash-cards/

Rao, S. C. M. P., 2018. *Dive deep into fungal overgrowth and digestive function.*
s.l., Shivan Sarna.

Raszkowski, R. R. M., Welty, J. D. M. & Peterson, M. B. M., 1976. The Amino Acid
Composition of Actin and Myosin and Ca2+-Activated Myosin Adenosine
Triphosphatase in Chronic Canine Congestive Heart Failure. *ahajournals.org*, p.
https://www.ahajournals.org/doi/pdf/10.1161/01.res.40.2.191.

Ruskin, J. & Vakuck, R. J., 2012 May. Vitamin B-12 deficiency associated with
histamine(2)-receptor antagonists and a proton-pump inhibitor. *Annals of
Pharmacotherapy* , pp. 36(5):812-6.

Saadi, M. & McCallum, R. W., 2013. Rifaximin in irritable bowel syndrome: rationale,
evidence and clinical use. *Therapeutic Advancement in Chronic Disease,*
March.p. 4(2): 71–75.

Seneff, S. P., 2011. *Sulfur Deficiency.* [Online]
Available at: https://www.westonaprice.org/health-topics/abcs-of-nutrition/sulfur-
deficiency/

Seneff, S. P., 2017. *Sulfate, A common nutritional deficiency, you're probably
ignoring* [Interview] (24 May 2017).

Silver Colloids, 2012. *The Herxheimer Reaction - Feeling worse before feeling
better.* [Online]
Available at: http://www.silver-colloids.com/Pubs/herxheimer.html

Singh, S. B. & Lin, H. B., 2015. Hydrogen Sulfide in Physiology and Diseases of the
Digestive Tract. *Microorganisms* , pp. 3(4), 866-889.

Sisson, M., 2012. *Why you shoud eat sulfur rich vegetables.* [Online]
Available at: https://www.marksdailyapple.com/why-you-should-eat-sulfur-rich-
vegetables/

Slazenger, S., 2015. *Inflammatory symptoms, immune system and food
intolerance: One cause – many symptoms.* [Online]
Available at: https://cellsciencesystems.com/education/research/inflammatory-
symptoms-immune-system-and-food-intolerance-one-cause-many-symptoms/

Spencer, T., 2014. *Structural Biochemistry Anaerobic Respiration Fermentation.*
[Online]
Available at:

https://en.wikibooks.org/wiki/Structural_Biochemistry/Anaerobic_Respiration_(Fer
mentation)

Stiefel, U. R. J. & Donskey, C., 2006. *Suppression of gastric acid production by proton pump inhibitor treatment facilitates colonization of the large intestine by vancomycin-resistant Enterococcus and Klebsiella pneumoniae in clindamycin-treated mice.* SanFrancisco , s.n., pp. Abstract B-1123.

Sutter Health, 2012. *Lactose Intolerance.* [Online]
Available at: http://www.pamf.org/southasian/risk/concerns/lactose.html

Sutter Health, 2012. *Lactose Intolerance.* [Online]
Available at: http://www.pamf.org/southasian/risk/concerns/lactose.html

Terzcak, T., 2013. *What is enriched flour.* [Online]
Available at: https://dontwastethecrumbs.com/2013/05/what-is-enriched-flour/

Thermo Scientific, 2012. *Test Principle ImmunoCAP Specific IgG4.* [Online]
Available at: http://www.immunocap.com/no/Products/Allergy-testing-products/ImmunoCAP-Lab-Tests/ImmunoCAP-Specific-IgG4/Test-Principle/

Titanbiotech , 2018. *Methyl Sulphonyl Methane (MSM).* [Online]
Available at: https://titanbiotechltd.com/methyl-sulfonyl-methane-msm/

University of Chicago , 2018. *How to Eat a low oxalate diet.* [Online]
Available at: https://kidneystones.uchicago.edu/how-to-eat-a-low-oxalate-diet/

University of Leeds, 2015. *Histology Guide, Epithelia.* [Online]
Available at:
http://www.histology.leeds.ac.uk/tissue_types/epithelia/epi_cell_junctions.php

US National Library of Medicine, 2018. *Lactose Intolerance.* [Online]
Available at: https://ghr.nlm.nih.gov/condition/lactose-intolerance

Vakuck, J. & Ruskin, J., 2004 April. A case-control study on adverse effects: H2 blocker or proton pump inhibitor use and risk of vitamin B12 deficiency in older adults.. *Journal of Clinical Epidemiology,* pp. 57(4):422-8..

Web MD, 2018. *What is sulfite sensitivity.* [Online]
Available at: https://www.webmd.com/allergies/sulfite-sensitivity

WebMD, 2018. *What is microscopic colitis.* [Online]
Available at: https://www.webmd.com/ibd-crohns-disease/ulcerative-colitis/microscopic-colitis

Weld, J. T. & Gunther, A., 1947. THE ANTIBACTERIAL PROPERTIES OF SULFUR. *Journal of Experimental Medicine*, 30 April, p. 85(5): 531–542. .

Wikibooks, 2014. *Structural Biochemistry Anaerobic Respiration.* [Online]
Available at:
https://en.wikibooks.org/wiki/Structural_Biochemistry/Anaerobic_Respiration_(Fermentation)

Wolters Kluwer Health, 2009. *methylsulfonylmethane.* [Online]
Available at: https://www.drugs.com/npp/methylsulfonylmethane-msm.html

Yang X, C. & D.C, M., 2006. Long-term proton pumb inhibitor therapy and risk of hip fracture. *JAMA*, pp. Dec. 27:2947-2953.

www.ingramcontent.com/pod-product-compliance
Lightning Source LLC
Chambersburg PA
CBHW060312030426
42336CB00011B/1009